LEARNING

Journals

LEARNING

Journals

A HANDBOOK
FOR ACADEMICS,
STUDENTS AND
PROFESSIONAL
DEVELOPMENT

JENNIFER A MOON

KOGAN PAGE

First published in 1999

Kogan Page Limited
120 Pentonville Road
London
N1 9JN
UK

Stylus Publishing
22883 Quicksilver Drive
Sterling
VA 20166
USA

© Jennifer Moon, 1999

British Library Cataloguing in Publication Data

A CIP record for this book is available from the British Library.

ISBN 0 7494 3045 1

Typeset by Kogan Page
Printed and bound by Clays Ltd, St Ives plc

Contents

Part III Practical issues in journal writing

Part IV Using journals more effectively: journal examples and activities

Preface

The content of this book is largely introduced in Chapter 1 along with a general introduction to the topic of learning journals. This preface represents a few notes on how this book might be read.

A book on learning journals might be looked at by those interested simply in the nature of a journal that promotes learning, those interested in the theory of how one learns from journal writing or those who want to write a journal for themselves for personal or professional development reasons. It might be read by tutors, who have decided that tomorrow they will confront their class with the task of starting journals and want to know what to do. From experience, there is a need for information about assessment. In the course of writing this book we have met many who are using journals with groups of learners, but who have yet to confront the problem of how to assess journals.

There are many ways in which this book might be read, only one of which is the cover-to-cover mode. While the chapters are arranged in a logical sequence for the reader of the whole book, it is possible to glean more specific information by reading a selection of chapters of immediate relevance. In other words, the chapters are relatively self-contained, and, in particular, that applies to the very practical approach in the last two chapters, which provide examples of journals and activities for use in journals. The cost of self-containment is a little bit more repetition than there would otherwise be.

With reference to terminology, we have adopted the term 'learning journals' but there are many alternatives that involve the same activity (see Chapter 1). The book contains much information and many ideas that would support those working as tutors or learners with portfolios. We have used a range of words with which to refer to the writers of journals – sometimes in accordance with context and sometimes to afford variety.

The book is particularly well referenced. It does not denote origins in deep academia. It is partly because there do not appear to be any other substantial bibliographies in the literature and it therefore represents an act of collection. It is also because the book is designed to be a practical support for those using learning journals for personal use or for use with others. Many of the references provide examples of how journals have been employed in different contexts and therefore they complement the material contained herein.

Part I

Journal writing and learning

Chapter 1

Backgrounds: some introductions to learning journals

Introduction

There are many different ways in which this chapter and, indeed, this book could start because there are many roots from which this exploration of learning journals has grown.

The chapter begins with a consideration of what a learning journal might be and the boundaries of the definition that are adopted for this book. The first section also provides a brief review of the uses of learning journals. We then ask 'why write a journal?' and we use some comments from those who write journals or who manage journal writing in educational situations to produce some enlightening responses. The next section roots the discussion in its past and present contexts. The past is history but towards the present, the interest becomes focused on learning journals as a topic in its own right in academic and educational literature. There is, too, a personal context for a writer's chosen subject matter and for this book, the personal context is more intimately related to the subject matter than in many other books. The section on the personal context describes how the book came to be written and how it relates not only to an academic interest in the human process of reflection, but to a personal life history of journal writing and, as is hardly surprising, a conviction of its worth. With some roots to the topic in place, we can begin to widen the discussion in the last section, towards an anticipation of the rest of the book.

What is a learning journal?

A learning journal is essentially a vehicle for reflection. Probably all adults reflect, some more than others, and for those who do reflect, being reflective can represent a deeply seated orientation to their lives. For others, the process would seem to come about only when the conditions in their environment are conducive to reflecting, perhaps when there is an incentive to reflect, or some guidance or a particular accentuation of the conditions. A learning journal represents an accentuation of those right conditions – some guidance, some encouragement, helpful questions or exercises and the expectation that journal writing can have a worthwhile consequence, whether at the end or within its process, or as a result of both.

There are many different words that are used to describe what we are calling learning journals in the sense that the word is used here. They may be called diaries, but not the sort of diary that notes dates for events, though they might do this as well. They may be called logs or learning logs, but they are not logs only in the sense of recording data at particular points in time or place. An example of the latter would be a ship's log in which data is written at fixed points in a passage. A learning journal is very likely to include some factual recording about place or time but for the sense here, it means more than that. Sometimes a learning journal is the same as a profile or 'progress file' (NCIHE, 1997) or a record of achievement, but it may differ. It may, likewise, coincide with many aspects of a portfolio in which a range of learner's work or evidence of work is accompanied by a reflective commentary. There are other words that have been or may be used to describe broadly the same activity as the keeping of a learning journal. Old terms are commonplace or common-day book (Rainer, 1978) which could be descriptive or might have a more constructive purpose. 'Thinkplace' or 'thinkbook', notebook and workbook are other terms that arise in the literature.

Precisely defining words seems to be unhelpful here. By learning journal, in this book, we refer to an accumulation of material that is mainly based on the writer's processes of reflection. It is written over a period of time, not 'in one go'. The notion of 'learning' implies that there is an overall intention by the writer (or those who have set the task) that learning should be enhanced. For this reason, the descriptive diary that never goes further than describing events is not part of the subject matter of this book. Within this generalized form that we are describing, there are vast creative possibilities. Some are described in this book and some are yet to explore.

However, we are not talking about something with a fixed definition and the essence of learning journal writing can be a little fuzzy at the edges. For example, while writing a journal mostly implies an activity that is personal and relatively, though not exclusively solitary, one form of journal writing involves two or more people who construct the same document. 'Dialogue journals' represent a conversation between two or more people, each responding to the other's entries, usually around an agreed topic, though, as in the nature of any conversation, the topic may shift and a new one may be introduced. Another example of work that may or may not fit our notion of learning journal is the autobiography. Many teacher education programmes utilize autobiography as a means of exploring students' pre-course conceptions of teaching, teachers, school and other concepts relevant to their professional development, which may distort their current learning. This form of work may or may not be sufficiently continuous in time to fit our definition, or it may be an exercise within a learning journal.

A part of the definition on which we have not yet expanded is the form of expression of the reflection. Most journal work is written and usually it is handwritten. A pen and notebook may not now be vastly more convenient to carry than a palm-top computer, but they are still cheaper, and for many people there is something more expressive about a favourite pen than a keyboard. Electronic journals have advantages, and one, in particular, is where parts of the journal can be communicated to another or others by e-mail – such as in the case of a dialogue journal.

In a similar way, verbal reflection can be recorded on tape – or the form of the reflection itself can be different. It might be drawn. In architecture or art, drawing or the exploration of graphic form over a period of time might be the subject of a journal and parallel ideas might be applied in music. While most of this book refers to written learning journals, much can be applied to other journal forms.

The subject matter of journals will be covered in many areas of this book. To some extent the subject matter of journals is implied by the three areas of journal writing that are covered in this book – journal writing in personal development, in formal non-vocational education and in professional education and development. There are large areas of overlap of likely subject matter in these areas. For example, few would separate personal development entirely from professional development (Harvey and Knight, 1996). Equally, professional or vocational issues may well emerge in a personal journal but are also sometimes of relevance to a student's development within his or her discipline.

Beyond the three big categories here, however, there are some surprises in the literature. While it is clear to see that there is no limit to the day-to-day subject matter of a personal development journal, there seems to be little limit to the subject matter about which journals may be written in the field of formal education. This book will discuss the use of journals in over 30 disciplines in formal education. These disciplines range far from the humanities and arts where the home of journal writing might seem to be. In a valuable manner, different basic subject matter inspires the development of different structures for reflection and writing and these different structures then can be adapted and applied elsewhere. Many of the exercises that are described in the last two chapters of this book have originated in quite specific applications.

Another major variable in journals is their structure. A simple personal learning journal may be no more than a recording of the features of the day with reflective commentary and consideration of the issues raised. However, an extreme example of a structured journal is also one most often focused on personal development. Progoff's 'Intensive Journal' (to which there are further references later) consists of 19 sections, many of which have associated methods recommended for their entries (Progoff, 1975). Between these extremes, there is wide variation, which is often defined by the subject matter or the purposes of the journal. For example, in formal education, journal entries may always relate to coursework – the content of lectures and reading work or entries may be required to follow a sequence of questions that are designed to structure reflection. Often, however, students who are guided in some of their entries are encouraged also to write freely in another section

The question of audience for the writing raises some interesting issues. It has two aspects. Firstly, for whom is the journal being written – who has decided that it will be written? Is there any choice not to write a journal? Secondly, who will see it – will it be assessed and seen by another in that context or will it be seen by a tutor who will ask only helpful questions to guide reflection to unconsidered issues? Individuals writing in a self-initiated manner may choose to share aspects of their journal with another for mutual benefit or purely for their own benefit. The coercion, the power and the nature of the audience can be major influences on journal writers, although, in the most rigidly structured journals, they may acquire a sense of intrigue and ownership in the process and none of these influences will matter.

Why write a learning journal?

Looking though the literature on journals seems almost to suggest that every time a learner chooses to write or is asked to write a learning journal, a different purpose for the process is given. In a previous review of this literature, we found that most journals were written for one or more of 18 different purposes (Moon, 1999a). In a reformulated list, these 18 purposes for writing journals are discussed in Chapter 3.

In this section we do not seek out the formal educational justifications, but intend just to give a 'feel' for the reasons why people choose to engage in this activity. We tackle this task by providing a couple of pages of the comments that journal writers and those who have managed a journal writing process have, themselves, made. These quotations are chosen because they seem, in many different ways, to articulate some of the essence of 'why write a journal'.

> In writing we capture a thought. We create order from fleeting metaphor, document meaning found in the world around us, place ourselves in time. We take something from inside ourselves and we set it out: it is a means of discovering whom we are, that we exist, that we change and grow. The personal journal has been used for hundreds of years to articulate the human drama of living and to explore new knowledge.
>
> (Wolf, 1989)

> Journals allow a reticent student to establish an opinion about a topic before being asked to speak about it publicly.... Journal writing turns students into active learners – it's difficult to fall asleep while writing! Journal writing also helps students to relax when they write and helps them to find their own voice and rhythm.
>
> (Carlsmith, www)

> I am an addicted diary keeper. I have been keeping a journal or diary... for almost 14 years now... This is no easy task. The act of writing requires the neglect of other aspects of one's life. With this huge price to pay, why do I go on writing?...

We literally write our own stories, simultaneously incorporating our own future, as we reconstruct our past.

(Cooper, 1991)

Now I had a boyfriend and, without realizing why, I wrote that diary to and for him.... One evening, without fully understanding what I was doing, I suddenly scribbled across the page in a large hand: 'LET MY PAGE BE A WOMAN FOR THE FIRST TIME!' and then, 'there is nothing but blank before me. I don't know where to begin'. In that moment, on that page, I finally met myself as the audience of my own diary. In retrospect I consider it the single most important moment in my life.

(Rainer, 1978: 31)

The aim of the journal is partially to individualize the undergraduate psychology course. It is described to students as a means of connecting the knowledge, concepts and ideas which they acquire from the course to their past and present experiences, thoughts, work, self-reflections; books or articles read; and other courses.

(Hettich, 1976)

Keeping a Diary
I try to observe my own experience
And discover that the more I look the more I see
But I do not know how to learn from what I see

(Joanna Field, 1951: 7)

When we introduced reflection, students often said: 'Yes, but what do you want us to do?'... Procrastination was common and it was typical for them to 'ramble'. But we found that growth was often a product of the ramblings, questions and explorations. One student offered this description: 'I just ramble until all of a sudden two or three words will fit together and key something. Then I realize that's it! That's where I'm having the problem!'

(Canning, 1991)

[Journal writing]... allows one to recognize, in writing, the natural thought processes.

(a student's comment in Wetherell and Mullins, 1996)

To some extent, we sense some meaning in each event as we live it. Much of the time, our response is so routine that the event adds little or nothing to our sense of our lives. Some events, though, carry a feeling of special meaning.... Keeping a journal is another way in which we may grasp a fuller meaning in these events and in the situations in which we undergo them.

(Cell, 1984: 221)

The act of writing is a great stimulus to creativity. When we are grappling with a problem, it is a common occurrence that in writing down our conscious thoughts on the question, useful associations and new ideas begin to emerge. Writing the immediate thoughts makes more 'room' for new avenues of thinking, new possibilities.

(Miller, 1979)

How... [do] I learn... I wasn't really sure.... Then, one summer, I discovered journals.

(Voss, 1988)

Education, as Friere noted rightly, can be used to free people or to domesticate them; when students write reflectively, I think they are being liberated.

(Sanford, 1988)

that is what my journals are about to this day. Moments of being in the world that I want to save. Pictures of the world that I have witnessed.... To reread the journal is to see oneself seeing.

(Grumet, 1990)

It is in the solitude of blank pages that adults can reflect on their life experiences, contemplate future directions, and come to trust more deeply in their own answers.

(Christensen, 1981)

Keeping a journal is a humbling process. You rely on your senses; your impressions and you purposely record your experiences as vividly, as playfully, and as creatively as you can. It is a learning process in which you are the learner and the one who teaches.

(Holly, 1991:4)

The data, though not conclusive, seem to show that journals helped students clarify their thoughts and enhance their ability to develop ideas.

(Dimino, 1988 – of nursing students)

One of the most engaging uses of personal student journals is as a mirror of the mind. In this mode, journals invite learners to find language deep within self to array one's hopes, dreams, disappointments, concerns and resolves.... The result is that students often express astonishment and delight at the kaleidoscopic self-portraits which emerge from the pages of their notebooks as they journey through a course.

(Bowman, 1983)

The purposes of the journal writing assignments are to encourage exploration and risk-taking by the students as well as to teach content.

(Hahnemann, 1986)

I've learned that the private fingering of ordinary experience can fill up notebooks as interestingly as musings on great events... My own diaries have outgrown the green strongbox I used to keep them in, and I've outgrown believing that I'm such a shocking character that they need to be locked up. They're a permanent part of life now.

(Mallon, 1984)

Journal writing holds before the writer's eye one image after another for closer inspection: is this one worth more words, more development?... It is this activity of regular informal, loosely-focused writing that helps a writer's thoughts develop and continue. In the academic world, where we teach students to gain most of their information from reading and listening, we spend too much time telling our

students how to see or doing it for them. That's not how I would encourage critical, creative, or independent thinking. Our students have good eyes; let's give
them new tools for seeing better: journal writing is, of course, one of those tools.

(Fulwiler, 1986)

In the concluding comments to his book, Hartley says: 'Finally… I would like to
recommend some specific actions that learners might take to improve their learning
and studying… to keep a reflective diary, making an entry at least once a week'
(Hartley, 1998).

We have made no attempt here to distinguish the quotations that arise from journal work in formal educational or professional development settings from those
that are personal. Sometimes those from formal situations are identified by their
reference to 'students', but not always. We make the point again in this different way
that that there is often not a clear dividing line between personal journals and those
'set' in a formal context. There is, however, one particular explanation for this blur.
It is unlikely that teachers would use journal writing and enthuse sufficiently to describe it in the literature, if they were not at ease with reflective, if not journal writing themselves. That journal writing in formal situations tends to be initiated by
enthusiastic and self-reflective staff has some consequences to which we will return
later.

The past and present contexts of learning journals

This section aims simply to set a context for the current popularity of learning journals with a brief review of past journal writing and of its sources in more recent literature. By doing this we highlight the more influential voices of the field at the
current time.

Lowenstein (1987) provides an excellent chronological account of journal writing before this century and demonstrates the range of purposes that have apparently
been fulfilled by journals. She mentions Japanese pillow books written by ladies of
the court and the subsequent travel diaries written by Japanese travellers. These diaries at times shifted in their content between dream and fantasy and apparently objective truth. Many diaries have been written for spiritual or religious purposes,
either as attempts to make sense of a person's relationship to deity or mankind, or
fulfilling a more established role in the ritual. An example is the confessional diaries
of the Puritans. Some diaries have had a deliberately community building function,
such as those of the Quakers, and many others relate to the records of lives or elements of lives lived which have been preserved for some reason where many others
have been lost.

Mallon (1984) organizes another account of diary or journal writing according to
the apparent role of the diary in relation to the writer's life. In addition to travellers
and confessors, he lists chroniclers, pilgrims, creators, apologists and prisoners.
Under each of these headings, he explores many. A concluding comment from his
studies is:

After reading hundreds of diaries in the last several years, I've come to feel sure of three things. One is that writing books is too good an idea to be left to authors; another is that almost no one has had an easy life; and the third is that no one ever kept a diary for just himself.

(Mallon, 1984)

A number of journal writers and designers of journals in more recent times seem to be closer, in their intentions for writing, to the notion of learning in learning journals. Tristine Rainer (1978) considers four of these to be of particular significance – Carl Jung, Anais Nin, Joanna Field/Marion Milner (Field is a pen name), and Ira Progoff. These four pursued their journal writing in different ways, in order that they could learn about themselves.

In the case of Jung, many of the discoveries that he made about himself were applied to his developing theories of psychology and psychotherapy. His book *Memories, Dreams and Reflections* comes close to an autobiography, but at the same time is a rich record of personal learning, reasoning and reflection. In one incident, for example, from his adulthood, he describes the resolution of a period of personal tension. In trying to understand the underlying causes he decided to examine his past experiences and, failing to find explanation, 'I said to myself, "Since I know nothing at all, I shall do whatever occurs to me."' (1961: 197). The first memory that appeared was of building miniature villages. He describes how he subjected himself to enacting the play again, making buildings with stones and mud, and as he did so, finding his mind clearing with 'the inner certainty that I was on the way to discovering my own myth'(1961: 198).

Marion Milner's writings are particularly interesting because, like Jung, she describes actions that she followed in pursuit of her understanding of herself. She describes her first book, written under the pen name of Joanna Field (1951), as 'a record of a seven years' study of living'. The aim of her study was to 'find out what kinds of experience made me happy'(1951: 13). The method she used was firstly to identify happy moments and to record them in detail and then to examine the records for patterns from which she could generalize. The book is written as a chronological account of the experiences and what she learns. The passage of her study took her well beyond only happy moments. For example, quite late on in the seven years, after experiences of disturbed feeling, she describes how she came to two conclusions:

'(i) The cause of any overshadowing burden of worry or resentment is never what it seems to be. Whenever it hangs over me like a cloud and refuses to disperse, then I must know that it comes from the area of blind thought and the real thing I am worrying about is hidden from me.' She goes on '(ii) To reason about such feelings, either in oneself or others, is futile'

(Field, 1951:140)

In another book, written a little later, Milner (now using her own name, and a practising psychoanalyst) records, in a similar way, a further personal project of learning to paint (Milner, 1957).

As well as the similarity between the work of Milner and that of Jung, that of Ira

Progoff is similar to both in its active stance towards self-awareness and self-development using a journal (Progoff, 1975). Indeed, Progoff studied under Jung for some time. The format of the Intensive Journal consists of 19 named sections, into each of which different content is entered and across which there is extensive cross-referencing. As with Milner's work, there are extensive references to the Intensive Journal throughout this book, and it is described in more detail as an example of a journal in Chapter 9 (1).

The work that Tristine Rainer herself did in developing 'the new diary' represents a very significant influence on journal writing (Rainer, 1978). The new diary draws from the work of previously mentioned writers and, particularly in contrast to Progoff, is very accessible and well organized. She introduces seven techniques that she then applies to a variety of different human issues. The techniques include making lists, guided imagery, the use of dialogues and 'unsent letters'. Versions of these appear in Chapter 10. Examples of the issues to which these are applied are personal problems, the discovery of joy, work with dreams, exploring eroticism and so on. She makes a feature of the activity of rereading journal entries, which can become a source of new reflection and writing in itself.

Beyond these more personally oriented writers about journal writing, there are some more academic roots. Hettich has written about the use of journals with psychology students and for the support of other learners (Hettich, 1976, 1980, 1988, 1990). In the early paper he refers to Allport's discussion of the uses of personal documents as a method of research. Allport himself is clearly impressed with the data that can enter journals: 'The spontaneous, intimate diary is the personal document par excellence ... In its ideal form the diary is unexcelled as a continuous record of the subjective side of mental development'(Allport, 1942: 95).

In the mid-1980s Holly picked up on another increasingly important use of journal writing in the context of professional development, in particular teacher education. Holly's book, which is found in a number of editions (eg Holly, 1991), is a succinct and 'down to earth' gathering of information in amongst a large literature of other discussions of the use of journals in this field. More seems to be written about journals in teacher education than in any other form of education, at least of higher education. There is also a considerable use of journals in nurse education. The use of journals in these forms of professional education is often related to their adoption of the notion of reflective practice. Correspondingly, in my earlier book, I speculate on why reflective practice should be particularly popular in these professions. Gender issues (more women), the interpretive relationship between theory and practice and certain professional vulnerabilities could be partial explanations. Chapter 5 elaborates on journal writing in professional development.

Another root from which journal writing has developed, particularly in the United States, is that of the proponents of writing as a means of learning. There are many ways in which writing can be linked to learning and the enhancement of learning and memory and this reasoning has been used to advance the cause of journal writing (Britton, 1972; Emig, 1977; Elbow, 1981; Yinger and Clark, 1981). This constitutes some of the subject matter of Chapter 2. Emerging from this line of thinking were two books in the mid-1980s that probably represent the best source material for ideas and methods of journal writing. The first, edited by Young and Fulwiler (1986), is a collection of papers about the value of writing of different forms in all disciplines. The second is also an edited collection of articles on the use of journals in all areas of the college curriculum (*The Journal Book* – Fulwiler, 1987). Beyond this latter book and that of Holly (1991) – mentioned above – and part of a recent book, which addresses journal writing and the use of critical incident analysis (Ghaye and Lillyman, 1997), the supply of books about journal writing seems, more or less, to have petered out.

One more root of journal work should be mentioned because it is certainly playing a part in sustaining and building the use of journals at present. It is the development of the theory and practice of reflection. The work of four writers tends to be particularly associated with theories of reflection in a fundamental manner. The first two are more theory-based. Dewey (1933) views reflection as an acute thinker/observer and interprets his observations from an educational standpoint. Habermas (1971) is an epistemologist and for him, the role of reflection is as a tool in the development of different forms of human knowledge. Schön (1983, 1987) instigated the wide use of the term 'the reflective practitioner'. The notion of a reflective practitioner has seemed to inject new life into some forms of professional education – often without a great deal of thought as to the real definition of reflective practice (Moon, 1999a). Kolb came from the traditions of experiential learning. The Kolb cycle of experiential learning (Kolb, 1984) identifies reflection as one stage of learning and is sometimes used to structure journal work (eg Wolf, 1980). In addition, we should add the contribution to reflection of the book of Boud, Keogh and Walker (1985), *Reflection: Turning Experience into Learning*, which itself was broadly based on Kolb's work. Either directly or indirectly, the work or theories of those cited above are frequently related to the processes or purposes of journal writing.

The personal origins of this book on learning journals

It is becoming usual for writers to tell the story of how they came to write a book (eg Boud and Miller, 1996). It is justified in a manner that represents some of the reasoning behind the writing of journals. Our perception of the world is based on the set of experiences of which we have been a part. Since we then further interpret the world through those perceptions, it is useful for a reader to understand some autobiographical influences on the product of a writer's mind.

I begin... and I begin with something I am learning as these words appear on the screen. We are clearly now in the land of the first person singular. As I settle comfortably into a style of writing that comes from many, many years of writing journals, I notice that the very letter 'I' seems to be a trigger into this writing style (see Weil, 1996).

I began writing diaries when I was 11. Looking at the tatty red notebook, it seems that I mainly wrote only on holidays to begin with. The entries are notes about what we did as a family – usually about swimming and sometimes deteriorating to days described lazily as – 'as usual'. There are no reflective entries, though I know that my daughter of 11 is capable of deeply reflective personal writing. Alongside my diary of that time, though, I have another notebook, this covered in plastic kitchen table-covering with bottles and wine glasses on it. It is a story I wrote when I was about 12. It did not start out to be autobiographical, but I know that that is how it became. It extolled the depths of feelings of that age and I think that that is where I truly began to reflect. It was easier, at first, to displace my musings to another person. The story certainly seems to belong with my diaries.

The next diary is a locking five-year diary in green. My current self does not know where the key is and I wonder if I will have to break in, but I find my hands feel for the tag and I almost watch them pull out the key. Pulling out the key is a habit of all those five years because there are five years' worth of close handwriting – my ado-lescence in 5 times 365 entries, beginning at age 14. I can now see reflectivity creep-ing into the first few entries: 'School was very much as usual today, but I was very much teased about liking Chris Collins (and I do). I wonder if he likes me....' Flicking further through the pages I come to an encoded area and I am pleased to find a list of codes. Adolescence must have its secrets (adolescence alone, I query). The information that I had been kissed for the first time was too sensitive to be dis-played in readable text, even in a locked diary. Thinking about my mother's horror two years later that I might have been kissing a boy leads me to think, even now, that there was justification for the code.

I open the red lockable five-year diary, which covers the period from age 19 to 23. I glance through the entries. There is one about going to a restaurant. I wrote what I ate. I recall that meal. It was a windy and wet night. Without my writing of the time, it is unlikely that that experience would ever have emerged. I notice another entry, this time on my 23rd birthday. John was my husband – the marriage did not last. I wrote: 'John gave me (extra!) a box of mint creams and a box of chocolates – I cannot imagine why – I cannot bear sweets for presents and wish he'd learn. I expect he'll eat most of them anyway. He keeps me neatly in stock and eats most of the sweets himself. I think it is mean and disappointing.' I do not suppose that I ever quietly conveyed my resentment to the poor man. If this were a true learning journal, I would like to think that I would have intended to take action rather than simply ob-serving.

The third five-year diary took me out of marriage and into what I have always felt was my true adolescence. It was then, not during my teens, that I broke away from the mould of my parents and created a fragile new self. I became involved in en-counter groups and a variety of 'growth' activities and reflection became a pillar of my existence. The diary is not complete. In June 1975 it stops abruptly because I at-tended a Progoff Intensive Journal Workshop in Edinburgh and began an entirely different form of writing. Attending that weekend influenced my life and, in itself, was a profound experience for the spiritual feelings that were generated by working with a group of people in that manner.

The example in Chapter 9 provides more information about the Intensive Jour-nal. I have mentioned the 19 sections above. In my bookcases, I have three or four fat tomes of loose-leaf pages in the 19 sections. From early on, though, the entries in the daily log predominated, often expanding into manners of working that should have been cross-referenced and placed in other sections. For long-term and day-to-day working, I have always felt that the Intensive Journal is too complex and that is why I have considered how it might be made easier for use. For short periods of time or for workshops, I think that the structure is very facilitative and powerful. On the basis of these thoughts, which have come to a head in tackling journal writing in objective terms in this book, I have redesigned the journal that I keep. I describe the new format in Chapter 9 as another example.

Over the years I believe that there were one or maybe two gaps during which I did not write for a time. I almost certainly wrote the equivalent material into letters to friends even if I did not retain a record of it. Over the years I have deliberately not shared what I have written. In one or two places among the pages of journals there are notes for the attention of others whom I knew, at the time, to be peeping. I feel a sense of intrusion when this has happened. On one occasion, at the bad end of a relationship, I faked a few entries, implying that I was having another relationship. Sure enough, the issue of this 'affair' arose in flames and the culprit truly indited himself. The lesson I learnt from that, though, was how difficult it was to extricate myself from my act of fiction. He would not believe that my entries were not genuine!

I come to the present. My 'brief' journal lies on the table in front of me, a small flat folder covered with maroon leather, which fits into my handbag. I have become more conscious of the learning aspect of journal writing as I have read papers in preparation for this book. I enjoy noticing when I learn something new about myself. From that point of view, I have great admiration for the learning projects of Joanna Field (Marion Milner). One day, when I have more time….

In addition to retaining and revamping my usual journal style, I have, during the period of thinking about this book, started another journal. I decided to try writing a project journal that would record my thoughts and reflections about the development of this book. It has been enormously helpful and again I present the idea as an example in Chapter 9. I would highly recommend the process to others engaged in projects that are not completely straightforward. Recording the inspirations and decision making that underpin the development of work seems to have made the process a deeper and richer experience.

This leads me to the last paragraphs before I pull back into more objective language. How has journal writing affected me and how has it contributed to my life? A journal is a friend that is always there and is always a comfort. In bad moments, I write, and usually end up feeling better. It reflects back to me things that I can learn about my world and myself. It represents a private space in my life, a beautiful solitude, the moments before I go to sleep just to stop and note what is 'there' about the day or about my life at the time. I think that it has enabled me to feel deeper and more established as a person, more in control but more trusting of life. On a less introverted note, I think that it contributes to my ability to write in general, and it underlies an interest in poetry and creative writing which awaits a quieter time in my life for fulfilment. In addition, I consider that journal writing is closely linked with the extensive counselling and hypnotherapy work that I have done over the years. It has been a support and a resource and a means of exploration, though I cannot say whether journal writing led to counselling or whether they both emerged as a result of particular traits in my personality.

The contributions from journal writing to my life have not come about through one or two entries to a journal. They have come over a long time. This represents a very important area of learning for me, the truth of which has only dawned as I have spoken with others who write journals. My view of the world, even what I learn from what I write in any one entry, is not 'truth'. It represents my construct of what appears to be truth in that moment and in another moment the learning may be different. Alongside the learning from the making of any one entry, I need to have the ability to put judgements on hold and watch how subsequent entries shape the same issue. That is when the universality of the learning becomes evident – or not.

There are other origins of this book as well. One that I characterize as the development of an academic and work-oriented interest in the topic of reflection is particularly important. Over the years I have worked with many small groups and in many educational situations – from primary school classrooms to classes for older adults in the skills of assertiveness. I have always been interested in helping people to learn more effectively. Around seven years ago I was in a post in professional education in health education. I was involved in the development of training for nurses and others with opportunities to educate for health. I became concerned when I observed the number of short courses that people attended which led them to do nothing different when they went back to work, and I began to build reflective activities and writing into the courses that I designed (HEA, HEBS, HPW, HPANI, 1995; Moon, 1996a). I was also concerned at the ineffectiveness of some national meetings and again designed ways of using reflective techniques to ensure efficiency and a more productive outcome (Moon and England, 1994).

In a later post in credit development in UK higher education, I was required to coordinate the writing of guidelines for the use of learning outcomes for modules. When, in a post that concerned learning support, I at last had the time to think about the implications of learning outcomes for teaching and learning, I found myself in an apparently conflicting position of promoting reflective methods in learning, and the use of learning outcomes. I wondered how I could be in the position of favouring a method that apparently promoted divergence in learning – reflection; and learning outcomes that apparently control learning in a convergent manner. I did find a resolution that seems, at the moment, to satisfy me (Moon, 1999b).

These interests in reflection were developing thick and fast in both a theoretical and practical manner and I felt I needed to know more about how reflection actually relates to learning. I looked at the literature and found it mainly dispersed into disciplinary or topic approaches. There was, for example, plenty of writing about reflection in nursing education and practice and teacher education, there were theories around and practices of encouraging reflection, but little consideration across all these areas. There also seemed to be strong implications that reflection is related to better qualities of learning (deep learning – Entwistle, 1996). The initial researches resulted in writing that culminated in my book on reflection in learning and professional development (Moon, 1999a). I was determined that – in addition to the theory, the attempt to clarify the nature of reflection across all of its educational applications – there would be a presentation of practical means by which learning could be enhanced by the encouragement of reflection. The final four chapters of the book on reflection have a practical orientation and the last but one is exclusively devoted to the use of learning journals. From writing a book on reflection in learning with a chapter on learning journals, it was but a short step to gather in all my personal experiences of journal writing and to contemplate, to research and begin to write this book on learning journals.

The layout of this book

This chapter has introduced the idea of learning journals and some reasons why this book came to be written. While this chapter has already begun to use the term 'learning journal', it is Chapter 2 that seeks the justification for the name. How do journals help learning? We consider some of the underpinning theory of learning and of representing that learning in writing that relates to the practice of journal writing. These two chapters represent the first part of this book.

Part 2 is concerned with the uses of learning journals. Chapter 3 explores the surprisingly wide range of purposes for which journals are employed both personally and in educational situations. Chapter 4 is concerned with the application of learning journals in many disciplines in higher education. The expectation might well be that learning journals only have a place in the humanities or other disciplinary areas in which sustained writing is a normal practice. In fact the literature provides accounts of the use of journals in over 30 disciplines and these are probably sufficient to allow us the suggestion that learning journals have potential application in any subject matter.

Despite the wide range of literature about journals in disciplinary contexts, the greater volume of literature probably seems to come from their use in professional development, particularly in teacher education programmes. Chapter 5 considers their role in these subject areas – in initial and continuing professional development, in institutional contexts and in the context of short courses. Although it may be difficult to separate personal from professional development, some accounts of the use of journals clearly relate only to the personal element, to which Chapter 6 is devoted.

Part 3 of the book represents the beginning of the substantial practical contribution of the book. Chapter 7 is concerned with the 'how to' issues – it discusses the format of journals; problems of starting to write; how to help those who seem to find reflection difficult; the conditions for successfully sustaining the writing of journals and so on. Chapter 8 takes on the difficult topic of the assessment of learning journals. This is a particularly important chapter in this book because there do not seem to be, in the literature, any other general discussions of the assessment of reflection that provide practical suggestions. While it may not always be necessary to assess reflective work, in many situations in higher education, journals would simply not be kept if there were not some form of assessment process associated with the activity.

The last part of the book – Part 4 – is more practical. Chapter 9 provides descriptions of ways of using journals under a number of different circumstances. Chapter 10 consists of a range of journal activities that can promote motivation, interest and specific forms of learning from journals.

Chapter 2

Learning from learning journals

Introduction

It is not easy to distinguish a descriptive journal from what we are calling a learning journal. The intention to learn from the journal provides the main difference, and using this criterion allows the inclusion of learning journals of novice writers who are finding difficulty in moving on from description, but who intend to learn. Learning can, anyway, take place as a result of descriptive writing. As Rainer (1978) suggests, people can learn to be free and to express themselves through simply writing. However, this learning might seem to represent a different type from that which occurs when a person writes reflectively. Reflective writing could be likened to using the page as a meeting place in which ideas can intermingle and, in developing, give rise to new ideas for new learning.

The literature on journals makes it clear that there is no one type of learning that results from working with journals. The paragraph above suggests that one somewhat arbitrary division is between the learning that occurs in the process of describing and learning that emerges as an outcome of what might be called 'thinking on paper'. Few authors in the literature seem to be aware of these different sources of learning when they write about their work. They are often more keen to evaluate journals on the basis only of a purpose which they have set for the task. McCrindle and Christensen (1995) and Dart *et al* (1998) represent an exception to this in their concern for the wider consequences of using a learning journal (see below).

Theories that elucidate journal learning

In general terms, there seem to be four main bodies of theory that elucidate the various ways in which journal writing might lead to learning. The bodies of theory are not completely separated, nor is there consistency within the area of theory. For example, in the study of reflection, the writers have come from different origins or disciplines, and tend not to have gone far outside their field in their literary research. Links between these areas of theory will be identified.

In the first body of theory we review the manner in which journal writing appears to 'fit' a number of conditions that are seen to favour learning. The second area of theory relates to reflection. Many who write about journals try to review reflection as a means of introducing their work. It is a nebulous topic with a very broad literature and multiple interpretations, and perhaps because many writers cannot grasp the whole field in a few introductory paragraphs, they grasp one or two significant names and base their discussion on those names. We have mentioned some, for example Dewey (1933), Schön (1983, 1987) and Boud, Keogh and Walker (1985). Instead of an approach based on a few names here, we build on my previous work in which I attempted both to 'grasp the wider field' and to take it further in relating reflection to learning (Moon, 1999a).

Journal writing and reflection have separately been associated with the process of metacognition – the process of overviewing one's own mental functioning, and this is a third area of theory described below. While metacognition would not appear to account for all of the learning that results from writing a journal, it seems to indicate a reason for some of the more general benefits to study that can occur (McCrindle and Christensen, 1995).

The fourth area of supporting theory in this chapter is focused on the process of writing – relating writing to learning. While much of this area of theorizing does not specifically refer to writing journals, it appears to have inspired and justified the use of journals for enhancing the learning of different age groups and across the curriculum (eg Young and Fulwiler, 1986).

From these accounts of contributing theory, this chapter on learning from learning journals moves on to speculate on the processes that might be involved when one writes reflectively in a journal. This latter section draws together some of the ideas developed in the three areas of theory and provides a basis for subsequent discussions on starting to write journals (Chapter 7) and the assessment of journals (Chapter 8).

First, however, we look at learning from learning journals by considering the way in which the nature of the journal task simply provides some conditions that are favourable to learning. We introduce this topic briefly now and return to apply it in a practical manner to the initiation of journal writing (Chapter 7).

Journal writing as a process that accentuates favourable conditions for learning

Journals favour learning through the encouragement of conditions for learning. Journal writing also produces good conditions for reflection and since reflection enhances learning, we shall not try to tease out the interrelationships but will regard them as a mutually reinforcing system.

Reasonably adept journal writing favours learning by **demanding time and intellectual space** (Barnett, 1997). The learner is forced to stop and think in order to write and in an educational or professional environment, such time for reflection or writing can be difficult to achieve by other means (Walker, 1995; Wildman and Niles, 1987). The very lack of time, of course, is a reason why journal writing can fail (Selfe and Arbabi, 1986).

In that time-space in which learners write in their journals, they are, by the definition of the activity, undergoing **independent learning** and the encouragement of independent thought is a means of enhancing learning. The learners are forced to be self-sufficient because there is no specific answer to any question that they might ask about 'what shall I write?', though there may be structures or questions that will prompt their writing. To the degree that journal writing is independent, it is also '**owned**' by the writer. Although content may be within provided guidelines, the essential nature of journal writing means that – to use a metaphor – the writer is at the wheel and is steering. Rogers suggests that 'significant learning takes place when the subject matter is perceived by the student as having relevance for his own purpose' (1969: 158).

Writing a journal also provides a **focusing point**, an opportunity to **order thoughts** and to make sense of a situation or of information. In training courses, even of one day, an opportunity to write reflectively can enable participants to collect their thoughts about a matter that has been discussed with a variety of opinions aired. They can relate the content to their own experiences or previous knowledge (Chapter 10).

The nature of the learning, once reinforced by a journal, may be more robust. Additionally, most, though not all, uses of journals involve the acknowledgement or the expression of **emotion or affective function** which is considered to be a more complete form of learning (Boud, Keogh and Walker, 1985). Rogers says:

> Self initiated learning which involves the whole persona of the learner – feelings as well as intellect – is the most lasting and pervasive…. This is not learning that takes place 'only from the neck-up'. It is a gut-level type of learning…. An important element in these situations is that the learner knows it is his own learning and can thus hold onto it or relinquish it in the face of a more profound learning, without having to turn to some authority for corroboration of his judgement.
>
> (Rogers, 1969: 163)

The emotion may be expressed in the choice of words, or, in a personal journal, it may be the subject matter of writing, or there may be an emotional release – tears or laughter that emerge as a result of the writing. Field (1951) tried to learn about her own behaviour initially by observing what made her happy. Storr (1988) provides examples of how a number of writers appear to have used autobiographical writing as a means of coping with or working through the emotional deprivations of their childhoods. He applies this principle, for example, to Rudyard Kipling, Saki, and with reference to journal writing, Beatrix Potter.

Perhaps one of the most important ways in which journal writing provides a condition under which learning is enhanced is because it tends to deal with **situations that are not 'straight forward'**. King and Kitchener (1994) coin a useful word for this – 'ill-structured'. They define 'ill-structured' problems as those that 'cannot be described with a high degree of completeness', that 'cannot be resolved with a high degree of certainty' and where experts 'may disagree about the best solution, even when the problem can be considered solved' (1994: 11). As examples, they mention social problems such as overpopulation. Other examples are ethical issues and the task that Milner set for herself (above). These are not problems where the educational goal is to find the correct answer, but the goal is to 'construct and defend reasonable solutions'.

King and Kitchener (1994) found that the ability of subjects to cope with ill-structured material is related to their level of epistemological sophistication, their ability to understand that what we know is constructed from what seems to be the most reasonable at the time. It is therefore provisional and subject to re-evaluation, and conclusions about ill-structured issues are drawn with account taken of the best facts available at the time. The understanding is that the knowledge of others is constructed differently and that their well-argued case can have equal validity. King and Kitchener worked with thousands of subjects over a period of 10 years to develop the scale of reflective judgement. The scale is largely based on the development of epistemological sophistication of subjects and their ability to work with ill-structured material. The writers suggest that the capacities of subjects who function at the top end of the scale are similar to those associated with wisdom. They indicate that the ability to progress in reflective judgement depends on educational activities that are provided by work such as that in journals. They suggest, for example, that students are familiarized with ill-structured problems or challenging issues within their disciplines. They should be encouraged to explore different points of view on a topic, to understand that there are different interpretations, to make judgements and to explain their beliefs.

In my previous work on reflection, I closely associated the work of King and Kitchener with reflection (Moon, 1999a). The developmental importance of encountering ill-structured material indicates that a problem in the expanding current higher education system might be the provision of more 'ready-made' material to students – handouts, lecture notes on the Internet. We 'tidy up', thereby, the training ground of material that is ill-structured, challenging and problematic and we remove a very important source of learning. Challenging students' learning in structured learning journals can help to replace this opportunity for important learning. Through encouragement, training or by their inclination, students can be required to write about the issues that are problematic to them or problematic within their learning, and for which a direct answer is not forthcoming. This challenges their uncertainties and acknowledges problems that need to be resolved.

We conclude this section with a comment from a nurse on her personal experience of journal writing. The comment beautifully captures her learning from the experience of working on ill-structured issues:

all the turning back and turning over and again. I felt I was pushing myself into corners and forcing myself to stay there until I'd worked out a valid response....

And then it got worse as I took it more seriously. Back in the corners again and this time instead of crawling around muttering, I felt I had to stand up and confront the corners. I did feel like bumping around in the dark. Then it began to dawn on me. I was refusing to see that it was me who had to switch on the lights. And the switches.... generally ... were just above my head.

Ghaye and Lillyman (1997: 74)

Reflection, learning and journal writing

We have mentioned some of the names that are most closely associated with the theoretical backgrounds of reflection. Dewey, Habermas, Schön and Kolb all took different viewpoints but their ideas are complementary. In my work on reflection (Moon, 1999a), I suggest that while it may appear from the literature that reflection has a range of identities, this may not be the case. It is possible to interpret reflection as a simple activity, a development of thinking that has associated with it a framework of different inputs, contexts and purposes that cause confusion for those who study it.

My account of reflection seeks the common ground not only between the theorists, but also in the manner in which ideas about reflection have been developed in different contexts. Those, for example, who are interested in the role of reflection in experiential learning have tended to see it in the context of the cycle of experiential learning and Kolb's work (Kolb, 1984). An influential development of this work is that of Boud, Keogh and Walker (1985) who significantly bring the role of emotion into the picture.

Reflection has also been important as a subject of research and application in professional development. Nurses and teachers and, in particular, their respective educators have been enthusiastic advocates of 'reflective practice'. Their reflective practice has often led them into the use of journals, or vice versa – the reflective professional chooses to reflect and write a journal – and a journal makes most people more reflective.

A context that is, more than others, based on reflective activity is counselling, therapy and self-development. Somewhat ironically, the word 'reflection' is applied to another specific process in counselling. Perhaps because of the lack of verbal correspondence, there is a relative lack of encroachment of the reflection theorists in this area. We return in later chapters to consider both professional development and personal development in terms of their wide applications of journal writing.

Beyond these specialized applications of the notion of reflection, it is also an everyday word and apparently an everyday action. Because my purpose in investigating reflection was to find ways of using it more effectively in learning situations, I considered it important to define reflection in a manner that takes account of everyday experiences. In those everyday experiences we reflect on ideas that are not 'straight forward', that are, in Kitchener and King's terms, ill-structured problems. We do not 'reflect' on the route from A to B when it is relatively familiar to us, nor do we reflect on a simple mental arithmetic sum. We have said that reflection in journals tends to centre on ill-structured issues and this is one way in which it improves learning (King and Kitchener, 1994).

In a tentative definition, based on all of these different applications of the notion of reflection in the book, I consider reflection as 'a form of mental processing with a purpose and/or anticipated outcome that is applied to relatively complex or unstructured ideas for which there is not an obvious solution'.

We have said above that what complicates the picture of reflection is the range of different purposes or outcomes that the activity of reflecting seems to fulfil. These purposes, in turn, seem to be more or less associated with different contexts within which reflection tends to be described (experiential learning, professional development and so on). The different purposes tend to characterize the apparent nature of reflection and it is no coincidence that the list of outcomes/purposes of reflection closely matches many of the purposes for which journals are used (Chapter 3 and Moon, 1999a). The first list is one of purposes. We reflect in order to:

- consider the process of our own learning – a process of metacognition – see later in this chapter;
- critically review something – our own behaviour, that of others or the product of behaviour (eg an essay, book, painting etc);
- build theory from observations: we draw theory from generalizations – sometimes in practical situations, sometimes thoughts or a mixture of the two;
- engage in personal or self-development (see Chapter 6);
- make decisions or resolve uncertainty. We have suggested that reflection is particularly associated with resolution of ill-structured matters (this chapter);
- empower or emancipate ourselves as individuals (and then it is close to self-development) or to empower/emancipate ourselves within the context of our social groups.

Sometimes we reflect in order to achieve a particular outcome. Outcomes may be actions or forms of self-expression. We reflect to order our thoughts in response to an essay question, for example. We may not be clear about the outcomes that we aim to achieve, but trust that by engaging in reflection, we will 'move on' our thinking. Meditation and free writing, which might be used as activities in association with journal writing, are examples of reflection where the outcome is not clearly identified.

Emotion, too, can be an outcome of reflective processes, whether this outcome is intended or not. In many systems of counselling, the discharge of emotion during a period of reflective counselling is seen as a helpful event. Consciously or unconsciously defending the self against the expression of emotion is associated with a blockage of the process of reflection. The role of emotion in journal writing and in learning from journals is an important issue that may be considered by some to be a threat to its use as a technique in formal settings.

The purpose for, or outcome of, reflection that is of greatest importance for this book is learning. We reflect in the process of learning, in order to learn or in order to generate more considerations upon which we will reflect more. In terms of the role of reflection in learning, it is helpful, at first, to say that learning is involved in all of the purposes of reflection that are listed above. It is on the basis of learning that we review something, or develop ourselves or build theory and so on. Despite the ubiquitous relationship of learning to reflection and in order to focus on formal contexts of education or on deliberate attempts to learn from writing a journal, it is helpful to list learning as a specific purpose of reflection.

Although it seems obvious that reflection is associated with learning, there is little research that relates the two in a more analytical way than the instructional approach of the experiential learning theorists (eg Kolb, 1984). The cycle of experiential learning involves a sequence of stages of observation – reflection – concept development/theorizing – and action (following on to more observation and so on). In the earlier book, I explore the role of reflection in learning with reference to the development of a 'map' of learning and the representation of learning. Learning here is seen basically as the 'taking in' of information which is then processed and subsequently represented in some form of expression which may be verbal – speech, graphic – a drawing, motor – for example, dance. This clarifies the idea that it is possible to learn effectively but if we cannot, or do not, represent that learning, there is no evidence that the learning occurred.

The map suggests the role of reflection in learning by relating several ideas. The first is that of cognitive structure. It was considered, on an earlier view of learning, that learning was simply a matter of accumulating ideas – like building a brick wall with ideas being added, like bricks, into the right place. This view of learning suggests that the teacher has a task of feeding the right bit of information to the learner at the right time so that it can fit into the accumulating knowledge in the right way. In the 1960s and 1970s, this model led to much thinking about the 'correct' sequence of instruction.

More recent considerations view the growth of learning as the growth of a flexible network of ideas and knowledge – the cognitive structure. It suggests that when something new is learned, the idea links into the network wherever the learner considers that it fits and this might be in more than one place. Fitting new ideas into the cognitive structure and thereby making greater sense of the meaning is the process of coming to know something. Depending on the way in which a learner fits ideas together, the knowledge may be similar to that of others, or idiosyncratic. There may be external guidance for the learner on how ideas fit together, for example through social conventions or the structure of a discipline, or according to a sequence of teaching, but in the end, we, as learners, are responsible for the meaning that we construct.

Learners who intend to seek deep meaning rather than surface knowledge (Marton, Hounsell and Entwistle, 1997 – see below) do not only take in or assimilate the idea in order to fit it into their existing knowledge. They are willing to change their existing knowledge – the cognitive structure – in order to accommodate the new idea (Piaget, 1971). If what is 'known' already is a strongly held belief, learners may work very hard to avoid changing their existing knowledge in the light of new learning that conflicts with the original belief. What is known might be, for example, their view of an acquaintance as honest and trustworthy. On hearing conflicting information, learners initially deny the legitimacy of the new information, and then might struggle to defend their existing beliefs before, eventually, changing their existing structure of understanding about the person. On this view of learning, the accumulation of knowledge is a complex but potentially and indefinitely flexible process.

Another important aspect of this view of learning is that what learners know already guides what they subsequently learn and how they perceive it. For example, we can only learn what we notice and attend to. What we notice and attend to is determined partly by what we expect on the basis of previous learning. Going back to the previous paragraph, people's willingness to have their knowledge and beliefs challenged, and their willingness to change their minds about an aspect of knowledge, depends on their openness and willingness to attend to new ideas. A characteristic of learning at higher levels is the requirement to reconsider one's knowledge in the face of challenge and correspondingly it exists as a will and ability to challenge existing knowledge.

The view of learning described above is that of the constructivists (Richardson, 1997). It stresses that learners construct their own knowledge and therefore they construct their own view of the world. It confirms the separation of teaching and learning because it stresses learning as the responsibility of the learner. Teaching is there to help learners to learn and another way of looking at teaching is as one means of facilitating learning. There are other ways of learning such as the self-guided use of resources. The most important use of teaching at higher levels may be that it provides guidance as to what is important to know about a discipline and the traditions of the organization of knowledge in a discipline.

We have suggested so far that, simplistically put, learning may be a matter of fitting new ideas into what is known already, or of reorganizing what is known and accommodating it to the new information.

In relating reflection to learning, I linked this model of cognitive structure in learning with the notions of surface and deep approaches to learning. Deep and surface approaches to learning were constructs that had their origin in Sweden in the late 1970s when a new method of research on learning was developed (Marton, Hounsell and Entwistle, 1997). Most previous research on learning involved varying the conditions of learning (such as type of teaching) and then setting a test to ascertain the effects. The new research involved asking students how they intended to approach a learning task, then setting them the task and looking at the results of the learning in a test. Alternatively the learners might also be asked how they set about the task in retrospect. This research highlighted the importance of a student's approach to learning, and this later became more closely linked with the learner's intentions for learning.

The Swedish research suggests that there are two types of approach to learning that have an important effect on the outcomes of learning tasks, and more significantly, on the success of students in their courses. The two approaches came to be called 'deep' and 'surface' approaches.

Learners who adopt a deep approach to a piece of work intend to understand the meaning that is being conveyed by the writer or lecturer. They intend to relate the meaning to their current knowledge and the meaning may be added to their understanding or it may require them to modify their cognitive structure – or what they know – as in the ways we have described above (Entwistle, 1996). Deep learning is probably automatic if learners are interested in what they are learning. As they seek further information, they are involved in the learning in a way that makes it a part of them.

Learners who adopt a surface approach to their learning do not have the intention to understand and to 'own' the knowledge. They learn because it is necessary and the apparently easiest way to learn seems to be to memorize the main facts and ideas (Entwistle, 1996). The learners are not particularly interested in how the new learning relates to what they already know, or in questioning it. If the development of knowledge is seen as a network, surface learning can seem to be unconnected learning where the intention is to hold on to the ideas sufficiently to reproduce the material.

In an important piece of work, the results of which have been replicated in other contexts, Van Rossum and Schenk (1984) show that the outcome of learning is related to the approach adopted by learners. Those who adopt a surface approach tend to learn isolated ideas which they cannot organize into a coherent form, whereas those who adopt a deep approach appreciate the structure of the ideas as presented and might have the capacity to work with the meanings to create new meaning.

Returning to the role of reflection in learning, my account suggests that reflection can be seen as a form of 'cognitive housekeeping' that facilitates the reorganization of ideas that occurs in deep but not in surface learning. Sometimes learners adopt an approach to learning by inclination – they are interested and want to learn for understanding – but sometimes it is the required form of representation of learning that determines the approach that learners will adopt. For example, if learners are required to explain something, or to respond to a thought-provoking question, they are likely to adopt a deep approach that requires them to use reflective processes.

On the basis of the reasoning in the map, I suggest that it might be possible to 'deepen' learning. Deepening occurs when learners 'rethink' or reflect upon material that they have learnt through a surface approach. This reflective 'cognitive housekeeping' is a re-accommodation of the cognitive structure that occurs at a later time than the learning. This process might be the basis of much learning that occurs in higher education where the delivery is largely through lectures. It seems unlikely that learners have the time or intellectual capacity always to be able to deep-process the learning from lectures, when, at the same time, they are writing notes. The 'deepening' of the learning might occur at a later stage when the ideas are represented in reflective discussion in seminar groups or in the writing of an essay that is more reflective than mere reproduction of ideas.

Relating this to the process of journal writing, we might propose that the learner for whom reflection is a familiar practice in journal writing might be more inclined to use reflection in learning, either in adoption of a deep approach, or in the process of deepening learning.

Metacognition, learning and journal writing

Metacognition is defined as 'knowledge and cognition about ... anything cognitive' or 'anything psychological' (Flavell, 1987: 21) and 'the ability to monitor one's current state of learning' (Brown, Ambruster and Baker, 1986: 66). Sometimes the idea of ability to control one's cognitive strategies is included in the definition (Hadwin and Winne, 1996; Flavell, 1987), though Prawat (1989) prefers to restrict the references to the control aspects of cognition.

Flavell's (1987) suggestion that metacognition has three elements seems to be widely accepted. The first element is that of person variables. These concern individuals themselves and their awareness of their own cognitive capacities. Other aspects of person metacognition are the knowledge of others and what Flavell describes as knowledge of 'universal mental phenomena' (1987: 22) – a general understanding of people's behaviour. Task variables represent the second element of metacognition. These reflect the nature of the task and the learners' understanding of how this should influence their strategy for learning. The third element of metacognition concerns strategy variables, the way in which learners go about reaching the learning goal. Flavell indicates that these three elements would interact in a practical situation. In a journal entry, for example, where a learner was reflecting on a task, the learner's knowledge of his or her ability to perform the task would automatically adjust the strategy chosen. This categorization might be usefully employed to structure journal writing where a journal is used in project development (see example 5 in Chapter 9).

Journal writing has been associated with improved capacities for metacognition (McCrindle and Christensen, 1995), and metacognitive capabilities have been related to an individual's capacity to study effectively or to learn (Hadwin and Winne, 1996; Ertmer and Newby, 1996). It might seem, therefore, that the development of metacognitive abilities may be a further explanation for the support that journal writing provides for general aspects of learning. Dart *et al* (1998) give some examples of metacognitive comment made by teacher education students in their journals. Mostly these short statements can be related to Flavell's categorization (above):

> I like working by myself, not worrying about other people letting you down, having different opinions.

> As a teacher ... I would accept students for whom they are and respect them.

> What are we doing? Teaching or thinking? Are we filling students with information about certain areas? Or are we teaching them to think for themselves?
>
> Dart *et al* (1998)

A number of papers discuss the importance of metacognitive knowledge in the learning process. For example, Paris and Winograd say: 'The central message is that students can enhance their learning by becoming aware of their own thinking as they read, write and solve problems.... A great deal of research supports the importance of metacognition in cognitive development and academic learning' – though they admit to metacognition being a 'fuzzy concept' (1990: 15). It is suggested that the greater ability in learning is achieved by a continuous comparison of the performance of cognitive processes with the goals that the learner is set to reach. The information is used to monitor or guide the learning strategies that are utilized (Weinstein, 1987). However, it also seems likely that greater metacognitive capacities also mean that learners are more aware of, or more able to define, the goals for their learning, themselves.

In my previous work on reflection in learning, metacognitive processes in learning are represented as the most sophisticated form of learning. I hypothesize the existence of several 'stages' of learning, with the earlier stages representing the events of surface learning and three later 'stages' representing what occurs when a deep approach is adopted. The 'deepest' or most sophisticated stage of learning is termed 'transformative learning'. The learning at this stage:

> involves a more extensive accommodation of the cognitive structure and the learner demonstrates capability of evaluating her frames of references, the nature of her own and others' knowledge and the process of knowing itself. The process demands greater control over the working of cognitive structure and greater clarity in the processes of learning and representing that learning.
>
> (Moon, 1999a)

It is of note that there are epistemological references in this description and that these accord with the higher stages of the reflective judgement model of King and Kitchener (1994) that was described earlier in this chapter. The role of reflection is suggested to be particularly significant in learning of this type. Ertmer and Newby (1996) see reflection as the 'link' between metacognitive knowledge and self-regulation: 'Reflection makes it possible for learners to utilize their metacognitive knowledge about task, self, and strategies during each stage of the regulatory process: planning, monitoring and evaluating.' The authors see metacognitive knowledge as 'static' and reflection as the more 'active process'.

In their research, McCrindle and Christensen (1995) link journal writing, enhanced metacognitive capacity and the enhancement of learning in a discipline. They propose a model of learning in which metacognition and a person's conception of the nature of learning determine the choice of cognitive strategy adopted for the learning task, and these, in turn, affect performance. They tested their model through experimental work with 40 first-year biology students, 20 of whom kept a journal and the other half of whom wrote a scientific report in the same time. Those writing journals were asked to reflect on the nature of their learning in the laboratory classes and there was an opportunity, therefore, for the journals to influence their metacognitive awareness. The results indicated that the journal writers generally performed better than the report group in the class examination. Their knowledge was of better quality and better structured. They used more advanced strategies for learning and had greater metacognitive awareness about their tasks. In terms of their conceptions of learning, there was a considerable difference between the two groups, the journal writers viewing learning in a more sophisticated manner. As a result of this work, McCrindle and Christensen conclude 'The provision of opportunities to deliberately reflect on their own learning can constitute a significant instructional innovation for tertiary students.' It would be interesting to know, in this research, how the journal writing in biology affected learning in other subject areas.

Writing, learning and journal writing

Writing is a form of representation of learning and a means of demonstrating what we have learnt. It is not learning as such and yet, in a powerful way, the process of writing leads to learning or more learning. While it may be relatively easy for teachers to accept the learning role of writing when they apply it to their own activities such as drafting and redrafting a paper, in class, many only utilize writing as a means of expression or communication. In this mode, it is the manner in which words convey meaning and factors such as their grammatical correctness that raise comment, not the learning that might have accrued for the student in the process. In some disciplines, such as mathematics, writing may hardly be used at all and this represents a lost opportunity. Even in subjects like this, writing can be used effectively to promote learning as Chapter 4 demonstrates (Selfe, Petersen and Nahrgang, 1986).

The value of writing as an important means of learning has been discussed by a series of writers whose work is often quoted in support of the use of learning journals in education. Richardson (1994) puts these different viewpoints in context:

> I write because I want to find something out. I write in order to learn something I didn't know before I wrote it. I was taught, however, as perhaps you were too, not to write until I knew what I wanted to say, until my points were organized and outlined. No surprise, this static writing model coheres with mechanistic scientism and quantitative research. But, I will argue, the model is, itself a sociohistorical invention that reifies the static social world imagined by our nineteenth century foreparents.
>
> (Richardson, 1994: 517)

Some writers try to unravel the relationship between thinking and writing, or more fundamentally, language and thought (Vygotsky, 1978). However, the way in which neurons link up to generate the learning that occurs during some forms of writing matters less in this context than an understanding of how to use the writing process to maximize learning.

An important variable that should be introduced here is the nature of the writing itself. Formal writing as it occurs in formal educational settings is normally not the same as the form in which personal journals are written – and it is significant that the latter form is closer to speech. In encouraging students to write journals, we are usually asking them to write in a form that few would have used in formal educational contexts, and with the diminution of letter writing, it may be a relatively unused language. In looking at learning from writing in journals, therefore, there is more than one variable in that: the language is different from that of usual academic language;

the learning from this informal language may be different in quality or quantity from that of formal written language.

The relatively informal language – termed expressive language – is described by Parker and Goodkin as 'comfortable, ready to hand language' (1987: 14). They suggest that we tend to use it automatically when in situations 'which are new, puzzling, troubling or intriguing' (1987: 14) and when we are exploring and thinking through writing 'in which a writer gets into a relationship' with an issue. Relatively few of those concerned with journal writing note the significance of the different forms of language used in many journals and other educational tasks. However, some do. Weil (1996) notes the value of first-person writing even at the level of the doctorate. Selfe, Petersen and Nahrgang (1986) worked with mathematics students who were asked in their journals to write, in their own language, about mathematical concepts. Among other findings, the writers note that: 'The act of writing ... in their own language and using their own experience helped students seal such concepts and problems in their mind' (1986: 201). Selfe also worked with engineering students, again encouraging the use of informal language to relate their classroom experiences to their learning. One of the objectives was to increase the overall writing experience of the students and an unexpected outcome was that their formal writing improved (Selfe and Arbabi, 1986).

With reference to school children, Parker and Goodkin suggest that the usual encouragement to use more formal educational language can set up a barrier between student and subject matter, 'making it much more difficult to generate commitment to the material or to develop any real sort of thinking about it' (1987: 16). It seems reasonable to apply this to any age of student.

The term 'expressive writing' was used by Britton (1972) in a classification of forms of writing in British schools. He reported that in a large sample of secondary schools, there were instances only of 5.5 per cent of expressive writing as opposed to more formal writing. All instances were in English classes. It is the expressive language from which other forms of language develop (Fulwiler, 1986) and there are suggestions that for many professional writers, it is still the form in which initial work on writing tasks is based. For many of us it comes in the form of scribbled notes, comments to ourselves and lines drawn between ideas. In the process of writing this book, the use of a journal as an experiment to aid the planning has, as I have said, proved immensely helpful.

Britton based the theory of his writing on Bruner's (1971) work on language and thought. In an often-cited paper, Emig (1977) also related the use of writing for learning to Bruner's work. She referred to Bruner's suggestion that we learn in three different ways – though doing (enactive), though imagery (iconic) and through representational or symbolic means. 'What is striking about writing as a process', she says, 'is that, by its very nature, all three ways of dealing with actuality are simultaneously, or almost simultaneously deployed.' She suggests that in this way, writing 'through its inherent reinforcing cycle involving hand, eye and brain marks a uniquely powerful multi-representational mode for learning'. In addition Emig argues that the involvement of both brain hemispheres implies that 'writing involves the fullest functioning of the brain'.

Once allowing the notion that writing is a powerful way of learning, the means by which this learning occurs become clearer:

- Writing forces time to be taken for reflection (Holly and McLoughlin, 1989).
- Writing forces learners to organize and to clarify their thoughts in order to sequence in a linear manner. In this way they reflect on and improve their understanding (Moon, 1999a).
- Writing causes learners to focus their attention. It forces activity in the learner.
- Writing helps learners to know whether or not they understand something. If they cannot explain it, they probably cannot understand it.
- Along similar lines, being asked to write the explanation of something can encourage a deep approach to learning in the manner that the learner anticipates the quality of understanding required for the writing (Moon, 1999a).
- Writing an account of something enables the writer to talk about it more clearly (Selfe, Petersen and Nahrgang, 1986).
- Writing captures ideas for later consideration.
- Writing sets up a 'self-provided feedback system' (Yinger, 1985).
- Writing can record a train of thought and relate it in past, present and future (Emig, 1977).
- The process of writing is creative, and develops new structures. It can be enjoyable.
- The pace of writing slows the pace of thinking and can thereby increase its effectiveness (Emig, 1977).

There are many other ways in which writing contributes to learning that relate to personal development and the ownership of knowledge that has been mentioned above. Both to summarize the links between writing, learning and personal development, and to conclude this section, we refer to Elbow's (1981) contention that practice in personal writing develops personal power which he describes as 'voice'. We not only quote these words for the valuable meaning that they convey, but for the many qualities of writing mentioned above that they demonstrate. Elbow's words struggle to capture an elusive meaning and to represent it to others in a creative process of crafting words, of focusing and explaining. Elbow describes how his students, working on journals and free writing, have developed what he calls a power or voice:

> I like to call this power *juice*. The metaphor comes to me again and again. I suppose because I am trying to get at something mysterious and hard to define. 'Juice' combines the qualities of *magic potion, mother's milk* and *electricity*. Sometimes I fear I will never be clear about what I mean by voice. Voice, in writing, implies words that capture the sound of an individual on the page.... Writing with no voice is dead, mechanical, faceless. It lacks any sound.
>
> (Elbow, 1981: 286-87)

The process of writing reflectively

The previous sections have provided some indications of the many ways in which learners learn from writing learning journals. Because our knowledge about learning is not very well developed (Moon, 1999a), much of what we can say about learning is hypothesis. This section is more pragmatic. The work on this section was initiated because it seemed that, for several reasons that are explained below, we need a clearer idea of what happens when someone writes reflectively in a journal.

The 'map of reflective writing' shown in Figure 2.1 is designed to suggest processes that appear to be involved when someone reflects in a learning journal. It is called a map because, while it plots the main activities and a probable sequence, we would not suggest that the sequence will always be retained, particularly when a person is experienced as a journal writer. The word 'map' has a sense of greater flexibility than 'model' (Moon, 1999a).

The map indicates a series of simple stages through which the process of writing reflectively about an event or issue might proceed and it suggests some elements that might be components of each stage. The map can be helpful as a guide for those who are starting to write journals, particularly for those who have little natural inclination towards reflective writing. The map can then underpin the teaching or coaching of the process (see Chapter 7). Furthermore, in indicating some main stages and elements of reflective writing, the model informs the development of assessment procedures and helps in organizing our understanding of existing assessment systems. We return to the issue of assessment and to the map in Chapter 8. The processes of the map are described below and references in the description are to Figure 2.1.

We start with the assumption that there is a **purpose** for writing a journal. This may be very general or quite specific and it may or may not influence the manner in which any particular entry is processed. A general purpose, for example, is to enhance learning skills or, in the case of a personal journal, to learn more about myself. A more specific purpose would be to enhance problem-solving skills for a journal used in science. Chapter 3 develops the discussion of the purposes of journal writing.

Purposes set for journal writing in formal education may not be clearly communicated to learners – or learners may assume different purposes to those in the tutor's mind. Teacher education students in Salisbury's study thought that the journal they were writing was to keep them busy, to encourage 'self-flagellation', and to provide a means of surveillance. As a result they attempted to provide their tutors with apparently appropriate material (Salisbury, 1994).

The map assumes that any stated or assumed purpose for the journal is an influence that may or may not guide the writing of journal entries. It also assumes that there is an often unstated supreme purpose implicit in the very decision to use a journal method – and that is to ensure that initial ideas are progressed towards learning, or at least towards being – what we shall term – 'moved on'. By 'moving on' of ideas, we imply an assumption that new learning is not an outcome of every episode of reflective writing, but that clearer thinking, or new or more ideas, may emerge that may enable the framing of further questions for reflection.

In a personal journal, written only for the subject, there may be no necessity to include a clear **description of events or issues** upon which reflection will occur. However, in formal situations of learning or where the journal is to be seen by another, a description is usually necessary. An event or issue may be 'one-off' or something that occurs regularly, and a clear statement or description helps to focus thinking in a particular area. In situations where the journal is to be assessed, it may be useful to set some assessment criteria for the description to ensure that it is adequate. These may refer to the general observation of the event or the issue (a). An example of a description of an event for a student teacher might be a description of delivery of a lesson that was particularly unsatisfactory. For a personal journal writer an example of an issue might be a relationship that seems to occasion stress. In addition to the general observation, there may be references to personal behaviours (b) relating to the event or issue (eg what did the student teacher do?). There may also be reference to personal reactions or feelings (c) and there may be comments on the context of the event or issue (d). The description itself does not constitute reflection.

Several established scales of assessment criteria for assessment of reflective writing or reflection include a category for description, but as in that described by Hatton and Smith (1995), this is not reflection. A description, alone, can sometimes bring clarification but generally it needs to be seen in formal journal writing terms as a precursor to reflection, but not reflection itself.

Reflective writing would probably always include a linkage between ideas relating to the event or issue and **additional material**. If this does not occur the process is liable to be self-fulfilling in a manner that does not involve progression beyond the description of the initial issue or event. Additional material may include ideas not previously linked with the issue or event such as relevant other knowledge, experience, feelings or intuitions (a) or suggestions from others (b). It may include new information, such as from a book or Internet source (c), formal theory (d), further observations (e) or other factors such as the ethical, moral or socio-political context of the event or issue. This list is not exclusive.

The map uses the term '**reflective thinking**' to suggest a kind of melting pot, the general thinking process that works towards the outcome of reflection – the learning or the sense of moving the issue on so that more is known of it in depth or breadth of understanding. By reflective thinking, we mean mental activities such as relating, experimenting, exploring, reinterpreting from different points of view or within different contextual factors, theorizing and linking theory and practice. We also use the term 'cognitive housekeeping' (Moon, 1999a) to imply the general reorganization of thoughts on a particular issue. There may be a situation in which one is aware that there is a linkage between several known ideas or facts and the journal writing provides some 'intellectual space' (Barnett, 1997) in which to sort them out.

The reflective thinking may lead to the required result directly, but there may be some **other processing**. For example, the resulting ideas may be tested in a practical situation, or 'sat on' for a while to see whether they are appropriate and their accuracy supported in other situations or by other people (**testing**). New ideas are often drafted once and redrafted in the process of **representation**. The act of representing material is a learning process (Eisner, 1991; Moon, 1999a).

Finally, for this journal entry, or this issue or event explored over a number of entries, there is a **product**. Something is **learned** or there is a sense of **moving on**. There might, for example, be a statement about an area for further reflection, or the ideas may be described in terms of questions.

Journals in formal education may be structured so that issues or events are reviewed, and some points of learning are drawn out. In other contexts of journal use there may be no encouragement or incentive to return to the entry to tease out further areas that may have arisen, or to test the learning. A more organic form of journal management allows reflection to roll on, as well as to reach conclusions. Points for further reflection are referenced and returned to at a later stage. The structure of journal writing that Progoff recommends is particularly fruitful in eliciting new areas of a person's experience for exploration (Progoff, 1975).

Figure 2.1 is drawn to suggest a cyclical process in which the ideas from one period of reflection are subject to reconsideration with the addition again of further ideas and so on.

We return to this map of reflective writing in later chapters, in particular to help learners who do not find reflection easy, to understand the process of reflective writing, and in the context of the assessment of reflection.

Summary and conclusion: learning from learning journals

Following the somewhat complex nature of this chapter, we summarize some of the ways in which learners might learn from learning journals.

Writing journals often creates the conditions that favour learning:

- through the way in which journal writing demands time and intellectual space;
- through the independent and self-directing nature of the journal writing process which develops a sense of ownership of the learning in the learner;
- by the manner in which journal writing focuses attention on particular areas of, and demands the independent ordering of, thought;
- because journal writing often draws affective function into learning and this can bring about greater effectiveness in learning;
- through the ill-structured nature of the tasks that journal writing addresses. Ill-structured material challenges a learner and increases the sophistication of the learning process.

Through their generation of reflection, journals provide an opportunity for a range of forms of learning activities – metacognitive, through critical review, the development of theory from practice; learning about self (self-development); learning to resolve uncertainty or to reach decisions; learning that brings about empowerment or emancipation. Sometimes the learning that arises from reflection may be unexpected.

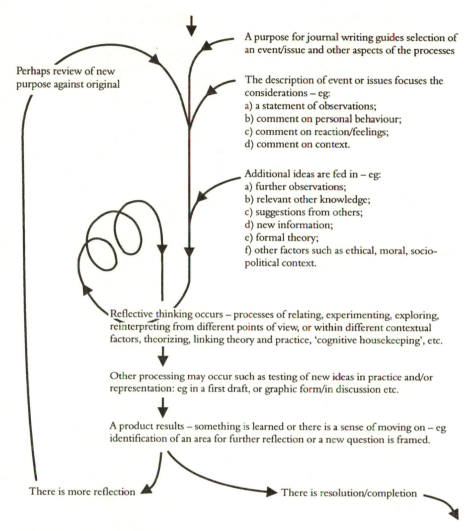

A purpose for journal writing guides selection of an event/issue and other aspects of the processes

Perhaps review of new purpose against original

The description of event or issues focuses the considerations – eg:
a) a statement of observations;
b) comment on personal behaviour;
c) comment on reaction/feelings;
d) comment on context.

Additional ideas are fed in – eg:
a) further observations;
b) relevant other knowledge;
c) suggestions from others;
d) new information;
e) formal theory;
f) other factors such as ethical, moral, socio-political context.

Reflective thinking occurs – processes of relating, experimenting, exploring, reinterpreting from different points of view, or within different contextual factors, theorizing, linking theory and practice, 'cognitive housekeeping', etc.

Other processing may occur such as testing of new ideas in practice and/or representation: eg in a first draft, or graphic form/in discussion etc.

A product results – something is learned or there is a sense of moving on – eg identification of an area for further reflection or a new question is framed.

There is more reflection

There is resolution/completion

Figure 2.1 *A map of reflective writing*

Journals encourage learning. Journal writing:

- demands reflective thinking and writing, which are associated with deeper forms of learning and better learning outcomes;
- is an opportunity to deepen learning that has been relatively more superficial – so that it makes greater sense to the learner;
- encourages metacognition, and this, in turn, has been associated with expertise in learning.

The use of a journal also improves learning through its use of the process of writing. Expressive writing which is usually encouraged in journals interacts with and sustains thinking; it provides a record of thought and maintains the focus of thought; it generates a 'self-provided feedback system' and in many other ways, writing can interact with and enhance learning.

We have viewed journal writing as a process that is specifically designed to bring current and new thoughts or information to bear on an issue or event in order to evoke learning or at least to 'move on' current ideas.

Part II

Journals: their uses and possibilities

Chapter 3

The uses of learning journals

Introduction

The chapter covers two different aspects of the management of learning journals that have a place somewhere between how we learn from journals (Chapter 2), and their more practical place in education, professions and living (Chapters 4, 5 and 6).

'Use' is a word with many meanings and we use it with two of them in this chapter. The first section of this chapter interprets the word 'use' in terms of values or purposes. In my previous publication on reflection (Moon, 1999a), I found that there were a large number of purposes for journal writing. These were not always identified at the beginning of the task. Sometimes learners were simply being asked to write journals with no purpose being formally specified, but at the stage of evaluation some of the outcomes of the journals were indicating new purposes for setting journals. For example, if journals are found to lead to improvement in the ability to write, then this notion might be developed into a distinct aim for later journal writing sessions. Different purposes of writing journals are sometimes better fulfilled in one format or another. The second section interprets 'use' in terms of the format of journals and we review some of the forms that journals can take. These two sections provide a grounding for the next three chapters on journals in particular contexts.

The purposes of journals

We have suggested above that the purpose may or may not be explicit. Most journal writing would serve several of the following purposes whether or not they are made explicit, and some of the purposes below would subsume a number of the others. Where the heading is the subject of a chapter in the book, the detail given is less – with the greater exploration in the chapter. In particular this concerns learning issues, and professional and personal development. Making purpose as clear as possible for learners is particularly important for helping learners to start to write, and in the relationship that purpose should bear on any assessment or feedback processes. The following is a list of purposes for journal writing and it represents a revised version of those in Moon (1999a).

To record experience

For perhaps most of those who write journals, the primary purpose may be to 'record experience', but then also to process it further (Brockbank and McGill, 1998). For some, the emphasis may be on the recording (Wolf, 1980) and this may approach the development of a log in its objectivity. Such recording may, for example, parallel research or project activity (Holly, 1989; Stephani, 1997). In many modern initiatives, experience is recorded in the past or present and accompanied by a reflective record that can take the form of reflective writing or journal activities. These may be in the form of portfolios (Burke and Rainbow, 1998) or profiles (James 1993), records of achievement/experience (James and Denley, 1993) or progress files (NCIHE, 1997). Some other examples of the use of journals where the emphasis is on recording experience include the use of journals to record experience in clinical (dental) situations that is beyond the requirements of the curriculum (Oliver, 1998). Another is the use of a log by clients in psychotherapy sessions (Fox, 1982) and in another example, students used journals to record their discussions with 'live' teenagers in a psychology of adolescence course (McManus, 1986).

To facilitate learning from experience

While some journals are primarily for the recording of experience, others emphasize the processes of reflection that follow the experience. This is the case for many of the journals in professional education and development, particularly those that follow either the Kolb cycle of experiential learning (Kolb, 1984) or the work of Schön on reflection-on-action (Schön, 1983) – see Chapter 2. Parker and Goodkin describe the role of language in first 'interpreting our interpretations' (1987: 176).

On a broader basis, journals that accompany field work or work experience provide a method of developing the meaning of experiences so that learners can relate their unique experience to established theory, or develop their own theory. Walker (1985) describes the use of a portfolio to support the learning on a course for those who would be leaders of religious communities. All of the teaching staff encouraged the use of the portfolio for which the aim was to record learning experiences in order to reflect on their implications for personal development.

To support understanding and the representation of the understanding

The use of journals to support learning is generally applied in most uses of journal writing and the role of learning in journal writing is explored in Chapter 2. Some examples in which the role of journals in learning is specified as a purpose are

Wetherell and Mullins (1996), who used journals on a problem-based learning programme to ensure the integration of learning, and Meese (1987) and Parker and Goodkin (1987) who have used journals to 'focus' learning. Ficher (1990) used journals to facilitate and clarify thinking and Wagenaar (1984), Hettich (1976) and Terry (1984) used journals in different academic programmes to enhance academic learning by linking it with everyday experiences of their disciplines. This might well improve learning through improvement of motivation and the encouragement of a deep approach to learning (Mortimer, 1998).

Others have talked about the way that journals are a means of slowing down learning, ensuring that learners take more thorough account of situations. They change the pace of learning (eg Jensen, 1987). Christensen (1981) considers that journal writing is a means of safeguarding learners against the push towards expectations of greater volumes of learning to be achieved more and more quickly.

To develop critical thinking or the development of a questioning attitude

It is also common to associate journal writing with the improvement of thinking skills. This category of purpose, however, is associated with critical thinking and questioning towards social change. Smyth (1989), in particular, focuses on the raising of social and professional consciousness as a purpose for journal writing.

To encourage metacognition

Chapter 2 mentions a number of writers who are interested in the enhancement of metacognitive capacities as an experimental outcome of journal writing. Others imply an expectation that learners will become more aware of their learning processes. For example, Mülhaus and Löschmann (1997) sought to improve the learning strategies of their students of German by asking them to take note of their learning in journals. Hettich (1990) introduced psychology students to models of thinking, and considered that with careful introduction, the parallel use of this material with journal writing could enhance student thinking. There can be a greater justification for knowledge of personal learning in situations in the education of educators, for example Morrison (1996), working in teacher education. Handley (1998), working with IT trainers, uses journals to generate understanding of the limitations of personal learning styles that might be presumed to affect their training styles.

To increase active involvement in and ownership of learning

Developing a sense of ownership of material is a condition that facilitates learning (Chapter 2). Writing a journal can have the effect of bringing knowledge presented as 'out there' into the ownership of the writer. It involves working with meanings and ensuring that the meanings relate to the current understanding of the writer. 'It thrusts the student into an active role in the classroom' (Jensen, 1987: 333). Tama and Peterson (1991) demonstrate this engagement in their use of literature to encourage reflection in student teachers.

To increase ability in reflection and thinking

Journal writing and reflection are linked in Chapter 2, both in general terms and in the manner in which I have suggested that reflection is fundamental to the taking of a deep approach to learning (Moon, 1999a; Stephani, 1997).

To enhance problem-solving skills

In some of the areas of the curriculum in which journal writing might seem less likely – in the sciences, applied sciences and quantitative disciplines – the value of writing has been demonstrated in the process of problem solving (Jensen, 1987; Grumbacher, 1987; Korthagan, 1988; Cowan, 1998a). More is said of this process in Chapter 4.

As a means of assessment in formal education

While we will argue in Chapter 8 that there are advantages and difficulties associated with the assessment of journals, there is no reason why journal writing should not be set explicitly for the purpose of assessment. It may be a less free-thinking version of a journal that results but this depends on the nature of the assessment criteria that are set in advance or that the learners perceive to govern their attainment of grades.

One example of journals as an assessment form is Burnard (1988), working with student nurses. In the context of education for returning adults, Redwine (1989) describes a reflective account that accompanied a submission for the assessment of prior experiential learning. This, in turn, would give exemption from parts of a programme of learning. In a more focused example, Fazey describes how she introduced student self-assessment diaries into the process of personal skill development (Fazey, 1993). Similarly, seeing assessment as a means of monitoring progress, Wetherell and Mullins (www) provide an example in dentistry.

To enhance reflective practice

As Chapter 5 will indicate, professional practice is a broad area of activity that probably includes most of the purposes of journal use that are listed in this chapter. On this basis it is interesting to note that it is in the professional development literature that the predominance of literature on journals lies. A particular reason for using journals in professional education is to enhance reflective practice. I suggested in the previous book that reflective practice seems to come in many guises and is therefore difficult to 'pin down'. However, it seems reasonable to surmise that reflective practitioners are reflective and understand how to think and learn from their experiences in practice and to apply and monitor the outcomes of that learning.

For reasons of personal development and self-empowerment

The use of journals to enhance and develop the self is the subject matter of Chapter

6. As a topic it overlaps in particular with professional development. Some would say that professional development inevitably involves personal development (Harvey and Knight, 1996). It is also the case that many of the purposes listed here could contribute to the empowerment or development of the self. On another view, the nature of journal writing means that there is an exploration of self and the personal meanings and constructs through which one views the world that is implicit in most effective journal writing (Christensen, 1981; Walker, 1985; Grumet, 1990; Morrison, 1996; Moon, 1999a).

However, there are some uses of journals that are directed specifically towards the use of journals to explore the personal world, such as that of Progoff (1975) and those who followed him. There is also a group, like Field (Milner), who set out to find out about aspects of personal behaviour to bring it better under personal control (1951).

For therapeutic purposes or as means of supporting behaviour change

One origin of Progoff's work towards development of the 'Intensive Journal' was in the context of psychotherapy sessions where he suggested that patients should keep a note of the 'events of their inner life' as they emerged during and between the therapy sessions. This appeared to have a valuable therapeutic effect and he extended it by 'drawing forward the inner processes' through questions and discussion (Progoff, 1975: 26–27). Fox (1982) used a similar technique with useful effects.

Used in the personal context, a journal can act as a place symbolically to offload the burden of unpleasant events or experiences, an 'emotional dumping ground' (Moon, 1999a). It can act as a way of working through difficult feelings, perhaps by writing letters that are not actually sent or for clarifying conflicts and working out guilt (Cooper, 1991). It was noted earlier that a number of successful writers seem to have worked through deprivations in the earlier parts of their lives through journals or other personal writing (Storr, 1988).

Reflection in journals can note or log behaviours that are irritating for the individual or for others and reduce their frequency or 'grip'. For example, a journal can be helpful to maintenance of a diet or other such behaviour change routine.

To enhance creativity

A number of writers talk about the relationship of journal writing and creativity. Journals may be used to generate creative ideas either at random or through focus on a particular project, or they can record and facilitate the development of the project itself. An example of a journal that facilitated the initiation and subsequent writing of this book is included in Chapter 9.

There are a number of suggestions as to how creativity is generated through journal writing. Milner's (1957) work on learning to draw suggests that one way is by taking account of the unconscious. Miller (1979) says that, as we write conscious thoughts, 'useful associations and new ideas begin to emerge', and writing the immediate thoughts 'makes more "room" for new avenues of thinking'. Through slowing and taking better account of the 'inner movement of our lives', Christensen (1981) suggests that intuitive elements of the self can 'break through' and give rise to creative insight. In contrast to these, Schneider and Killick (1998) approach the same subject matter from the angle of creative writing. They suggest that by using journals and self-discovery exercises (which they include), readers can find ease in writing from personal experience and thereby may improve their creative writing skills.

To improve writing

The improvement of writing is one of the more common explicit purposes for journal writing in formal situations (eg Brodsky and Meagher, 1987). There are a number of reports on the improvement of writing that has followed use of journals. For example, Jensen (1987) noted that physics students who wrote journals improved in their ability to write essays in a fluent manner. However, in journal writing, 'fluency can ... become gush'. Berthoff (1987: 14) points out the importance of maintaining fluency within the bounds of a structure that makes it productive. The improvement of writing ability may sometimes result from the opportunity that journal writing provides for integrating everyday language into more academic forms (Parker and Goodkin, 1987; Macrorie, 1970).

To improve or give 'voice'; as a means of self-expression

Some learners are not as able as others at self-expression. Journals provide a means of enabling them to express themselves in an alternative manner. There are different ways of learning and of expressing that learning. Some have much to express, but are not in suitable social or emotionally suitable situations for that expression. Journal writing is an alternative voice. Craig contrasts finding a voice of one's own with finding a voice 'that we think is proper to share with other people' and notes that it is then that 'we often lose our own voice' (Dillon, 1983). A slightly different view of self-expression is that journals increase active involvement in learning (Bowman, 1983).

To foster communication and to foster reflective and creative interaction in a group

Many talk about the use of interaction as a means of facilitating journal writing for individuals and there is literature on dialogue journals that are shared by two or more people (see later). However, some writers have mentioned a purpose of journal writing to be to facilitate the interaction within a group (Walker, 1985) and Hickman describes the development at what might be the extremes of journal writing – the office log to 'maintain communication and continuity' (1987: 391). In a number of evaluations of the use of journals in classroom situations for other purposes, there are incidental comments that students seem more willing to interact in class as a result of their writing.

To support planning and progress in research or a project

Journals may be concerned with quite specific issues – such as the work in one discipline in formal education. They may focus on one piece of work in which the writer is engaged at the time or is planning – such as a research project, a forthcoming event or trip (Holly, 1989). In this context, they become a repository of ideas, plans and thoughts that can greatly enhance the final product or the specific planning of the product. Perhaps the significant difference that the use of a journal during planning makes is that it encourages the practitioner to see planning as a process that occurs over a period of time instead of on one occasion. Ideas can be put down and modified or abandoned – the material is generally mulled over for a while and given time to settle into its most promising format.

As a means of communication between a learner and another

A general comment in a number of papers is that a sometimes unexpected outcome of asking students to write journals is that staff learn much more about their students as people and as learners (eg Wetherell and Mullins, 1996). The staff learn also about the students' perception of the course itself. In some situations a major purpose of the journal is to maintain the contact between a tutor or mentor and a student who may be in a location at some distance. An example of a use like this is where teaching students are involved in teaching practice in schools at some distance from the university. E-mail instead of pen and paper is used in this situation for communication (eg weekly 'chunks' of journal are transmitted from student to tutor who then has an opportunity to comment on the material and transmit the comment (Parnell, 1998).

A more equalized way of using dialogue between tutor and student is the dialogue journal format that is described below.

Forms of journal writing

This section again represents a modified version of similar material in my account of reflection (Moon, 1999a).

Journals come in any shape or size or form. They exist as the five-year diary with prescribed space for each day, they could exist as yellow sticky notes stuck on the walls of a room, or they exist not on paper at all. They may be in electronic form on audio or videotape or in a word processed format and, no doubt, they have been written on stone. The possibilities are as broad as the imagination of the writer – or of the person who has set journal writing as a task. However, a more significant factor for the learning result of journal writing is the internal structure of a journal. Writing, for example, might result from the stimulus of an exercise or a question posed, rather than only existing in the free-flowing form which is initiated directly by the writer. We explore here some of the more usual formats of journals and why particular formats might be chosen. There are three major divisions in this discussion. They represent the relatively unstructured journal, and those that are structured in some way and are written by individuals, and dialogue journals that are a form of written conversation between two or more people. The difference between structured and unstructured forms of journal is somewhat arbitrary and there is no reason why a journal should not start structured and then become unstructured as the learner gains more experience of writing. Indeed, while the structure may be helpful in early stages of writing, the big leap in improvement and satisfaction from journal writing is often when the structure is thrown out. Sometimes a structure is provided as an option that the writers may discard if they do not need the support that structure provides.

More or less unstructured forms

It is questionable whether any form of journal in a formal learning situation is truly unstructured. Any journal that will be overseen by another in authority is likely to be structured in accordance with the perceived expectations of the overseer. This hidden curriculum is of no mean significance as a structural influence.

Free writing and reflecting. The subject matter and content of the journal are more or less free writing, with no constraints on subject matter or the format of the writing – though there may be a requirement that is self-imposed or is imposed from elsewhere that the writer writes regularly.

Structured forms

By 'structure' we mean any imposed constraint on the way in which a journal is written. Structure can help students to obtain greater benefit from the journal. It can ensure that the learners reflect on the appropriate issues and can help them to 'move on' in their reflection and their learning. One form of structure may be the instruction to follow the events in reflective writing identified on the map of reflective writing (see Chapter 7). This will tend to prevent both rambling and 'going around in circles', both of which are less likely if the writers know the components that are expected in their writing – understanding, for example, that they must go beyond the stage of description.

Structure may come in the form of themes for the form of writing – such as autobiography or recording that relates to a project or issue.

Autobiographical writing. There is an autobiographical element to the writing, perhaps in the way that previous events are related to the current time (eg as in Progoff, 1975). Such a form of writing may accompany a portfolio, providing a commentary on the materials in terms of personal development.

Double entry journals. In this type of journal, the recording of experience is first made in a descriptive manner. At a later time the writer reflects and writes further on the initial written account, drawing conclusions from it or at least 'moving it on'. This further writing may be spatially arranged alongside the original, sometimes on the opposite page to it.

Structure is given as exercises. Some journals are substantially based on the provision of set activities or exercises such as those that are included in the last two chapters of this book. There may, in addition, be some free writing.

Structure is given in the form of questions for response or guidance as to issues to be covered. A sequence of questions provides prompts that guide the learner to cover particular or the appropriate areas of material. The sequence may mirror that in the map of reflective writing (Figure 2.1). The questions provided by Johns (1994) are an example here.

The journal is used to accompany other learning and the structure is determined by the other learning. The other learning may be a programme of learning or it may be, for example, a research project or placement. The journal may be written in the planning stages if it accompanies a project. The entries may underpin reflection on what actual topic to choose for investigation as well as reflection on the events of the actual development. If the 'other learning' is a programme of learning, the learner may be asked to reflect, for example, on set reading, the content of lectures or seminars (Chapter 4).

A journal format is used where the structure is provided within the journal itself. In this case the writers choose how to work within the set structure. Progoff's Intensive Journal is an example (see Chapter 6). In this case, the writers start writing in one section and move to another section, guided by the emerging themes as they work, or guided by what they want to explore. In the Intensive Journal there are suggested methods of working in the different sections.

Profiles or portfolios. There is another group of 'life accounts' that are not usually called 'journals', but can have the same effect. Portfolios tend to include other documents alongside reflective writing that summarizes and interrelates the document content. There may be other than written accounts included, such as graphic material, stories or poetry.

Profiles or portfolios are particularly common in professional development settings (Chapter 5), in the accreditation of prior learning, in fieldwork and placements, and they are increasingly being used as a means of assessment in discipline-based higher education.

Dialogue journals

We expand on the topic of dialogue journals here because the other forms of journal writing will be described in later chapters. Dialogue journals are different from individually written journals in that they encourage the exchange and development of ideas between two or more writers. They can be like the exchange of letters where the letter content is reflective. One writer starts, usually with a comment or a set of thoughts, and the journal with its entry is passed on to another who responds to the first, usually taking the ideas further, or adding new information. There are examples of this method in 'open' situations or set in a context with the subject matter focused on the issues of that context.

Dialogue journals seem to have had their origins in school settings with young children corresponding with their teachers in the 1980s (Staton *et al*, 1988), but their use is described in a number of contexts in more recent literature. These tend still to be in the teaching literature. Examples of their use are between professional teachers engaging in research of their practice (Roderick and Berman, 1984; Roderick, 1986) and between teacher educators and teaching students (Staton *et al*, 1988).

The literature on dialogue journals tends to make great claims for their advantages, but the purposes of their uses are not always very clear. Where they are used between an authority and a student, the former can steer the reflection of the latter in the conversation and the interaction is probably not unlike a tutorial. However, where the dialogue is between equals, the slow pace can have an effect of deepening thinking and learning and of allowing time for unexpected thoughts to contribute to the dialogue.

The modern parallel of the dialogue journal is the e-mail conversation in newsgroups. As these groups tend to demonstrate, there is a need for someone to take on a role of managing a discussion so that it retains a focus or a stream, and perhaps of summarizing it from time to time. An interesting issue, which applies to any forms of journal that are word-processed, is whether the nature of the writing process is the same as that on paper, or different. The speed of writing on a screen may be an initial difference.

Chapter 4

Journals in teaching and learning in higher education

Introduction

This chapter considers the applications of learning journals in formal educational settings. While the focus is higher education, much could apply also to the schools' situation. The chapter deals with journals in subjects or disciplines mainly other than those in professional or vocational subjects which are covered in the next chapter. There is a large overlap in the two chapters, partly because the notion of reflection and reflective practice from professional education is being drawn into the currency of thinking in general higher education (eg Barnett, 1997).

The chapter is divided into two parts – a short part and a longer part. The short part focuses on learning journals and reflective writing in more general activities of higher education that are not related specifically to a discipline – for example in the accreditation of prior learning as a result of experience. The longer section reviews the place of learning journals in the context of learning in the disciplines in higher education. Within these two sections, there will be many different examples.

General applications of learning journals in higher education

In some of the examples below where portfolios are mentioned, there is little distinction between the journal and forms of portfolio. They both rely on reflective writing which links theory, experience and observation of real situations and represent a collection of material over time.

Records of achievement or progress files

Records of achievement may simply be a series of brief details about achievements and experiences that are useful when it comes to writing curriculum vitae or attending an interview. However, they can be more, and this is implied in the term 'progress files' adopted by the Dearing Review (NCIHE, 1997). The record can be supplemented by a process of reflection on progress towards goals beyond the programme of learning, or on the ways in which learning from various parts of the programme interrelate or, perhaps, on the learning from leisure activities or part-time work situations.

Fieldwork or placements

Reflective writing, often in journals, is increasingly used as a means of accounting for and realizing learning in fieldwork, placements and in work experience. While it is generally recognized that students gain from the opportunity to engage in such experiences, the learning can be so varied and incoherent that it is difficult for the student to articulate it and apply it to other situations. Asking for written reflective accounts or journals either that are unstructured or that are structured in order to focus attention on particular aspects of the experience seems to be helpful. Students may have the opportunity to do work-experience modules which have a basis of reflective writing (eg Houghton, 1998). A variation on this theme in a practical setting, where some learning is formalized, is the use of journals to record incidental learning. An example of this is where dental students in clinics record the wealth of personal and incidental learning (Oliver, 1998). This might have particular relevance in situations where the stipulated learning is described in terms of competencies or national vocational qualifications.

Research or project journals

We have suggested earlier that journals can be a helpful adjunct to project work, forming a location for conventional activities such as the logging of events but also for the recording of deliberations over initial ideas, decision processes and reflection on progress. This process can be particularly useful where a number of people are involved in the work. It can then also have a focus of coordinating the group and of ensuring appropriate information flow (Hickman, 1987).

Career management

There are other projects undertaken by other students than those in the academic context. Learning career-seeking skills, learning employability skills, searching for a post and performing in interview form a project that spans most of the years of a degree. It is motivating and helpful if the activities are integrated. A journal, similar to the research or project journal, provides a location for noting achievements or experiences (eg the learning of skills) for deliberation and planning, and brings coherence to the process (NICEC, 1998).

Lecture journals

The lecture journal is a general method of journal use that can cut across all disciplines in formal education and can be used alone or as a component of a journal. One of the problems with the traditional lecture method is that in its usual form it may not provide the time during which learners can think about its content and relate that to previous learning or experience. Students also require to take notes that further cut down the opportunity for deep learning (Chapter 2). It is probably fair to say that most students collect the notes from the day's classes and file them away for later reference. A lecture journal, however, in which they reflect on the content of a lecture, provides the opportunity to deepen and thereby to improve the quality of learning. There can be variations on the theme. Students might, for example, be asked to formulate a series of questions that arise from the content of the lecture or to record a conversation with another about the lecture.

The development of writing skills

The topic of skills for employability is a concern for higher education at present. Writing is an important form of communication and, within constraints, features in most – but not all – disciplines. Journal writing does seem to improve written self-expression and, on this basis, provides a means of bringing writing into disciplines such as mathematics, where it might not normally feature. As the second section in this chapter, however, indicates, there are other reasons for instituting journals within disciplines such as mathematics.

In adult education or for those returning to education

Because journals are a means of identifying, raising awareness of, and accounting for learning, they have value for those in adult education or who are returning to education (Christensen, 1981). In this way also, journals have many roles to play in lifelong learning. Redwine (1989) has been mentioned. She describes the use of reflective autobiographical writing with students attending a ten-day orientation seminar prior to engagement in a degree programme based on distance learning. She identifies a number of roles that the writing fulfils. It is cathartic, helping students to bring to the fore and to deal with parts of their life histories – 'adults enter or re-enter the educational cycle with needs and characteristics that are very different from those of 18–22 year olds' (1989: 89). The shared writing develops group support that can persist and the task underpins the development of claims for credit for prior learning.

Journals in the disciplines

While subject groups and headings are used to organize the content of this section, many of the techniques can be applied in other disciplinary contexts. Similarly, across the accounts below, practically all purposes for writing journals (Chapter 3) are represented explicitly or as an outcome.

The sciences, engineering and mathematics

This is a group of subjects in which journal writing might appear not to have a place. However, among a relatively few accounts in the literature, there are clear indications of the manner in which journal writing can facilitate learning and help with writing and there are some descriptions of useful techniques.

Perhaps the most helpful reports are those that are experimental. Selfe, Petersen and Nahrgang (1986) studied the manner in which journal writing could help **mathematics** students. Initially their intention was to compare the test grades of a group that was asked to write journals with another group using traditional methods. They found, however, that the influence of journal writing was more subtle The general finding in the initial investigation was that journal writing was no better or worse than activities involving testing or quizzes at promoting learning. On a subsequent more subtle investigation, journals appeared to facilitate learning in a number of ways. By allowing them to think in a manner that was their own and to use their own language, the students were able to develop personal conceptual definitions that were much more understandable than technical definitions. The concrete nature of this thinking facilitated comprehension and application of abstract concepts and they began to evaluate or appreciate the usefulness of the concepts. The other two effects relate to the ability to solve problems. There was evidence in the writing that students were recording strategies that they found helpful in problem solving. Furthermore, in writing about problems instead of just working on calculation, they were coming to solutions through the writing. An excerpt from the writing of one student illustrates well the last point: 'I see nothing in common with the three functions except that the derivative has a power of N–1 just like all the other derivatives have. Oh – wait a sec, now I see how you did it. You took the derivative of the first term and …' (Selfe, Petersen and Nahrgang, 1986: 200). It is interesting to see the same process evident in the writing of much younger students (age 11) cited by Mayher, Lester and Pradl (1983).

Selfe worked also with **engineering** students (Selfe and Arbabi, 1986), with a primary intention of introducing more writing into the course. The students, in a structural analysis and design class, were asked to write at least a page a week on their experiences of the course. While their initial reaction was negative, and for a few (around 10 per cent) it remained negative, most found that 'it helped … (them to) … clarify their thoughts, work out strategies for solving engineering problems, understand the important aspects of the structures course and identify areas in which they needed more help' (1986: 185). In contrast to a control group, those who had written in journals wrote final reports that 'were generally more coherent, organized and complete with better description of methods used to solve engineering problems.' Instructors also felt much more informed about their students' processes of learning. Gibbs (1988) describes the use of journals in engineering in a somewhat similar manner.

Two examples of journal writing in **physics** broadly parallel the observations above. Jensen (1987) describes the use of journals initially in order to improve writing among physics students. His students wrote on assigned topics at the beginning, in the middle or at the end of lecture sessions for seven or eight minutes and they were encouraged to reflect personally. Some of the topics were: 'Explain to your mother why water stays in a pail when swung in a vertical circle around your head' or 'Discuss the net effect of leaving the fridge door open'. Jensen observes that the writing was initially formal and textbook-like and then became freer, exploring and extrapolating. Jensen suggests that the value seems not so much that the students had the opportunity to write, but that they were 'thinking on paper'. It is worth reiterating a comment in Chapter 2 suggesting that the requirement to be able to explain seems likely to encourage a deep approach to learning.

Grumbacher (1987) focused on the ability of physics students to solve problems. She observed the writing processes of students whom she considered to be good problem solvers. They articulate the problems clearly, use visualization and verbalization in the solving and they are aware of the relative appropriateness of their responses. More significantly 'they use their learning logs to synthesize their new knowledge about physics with their prior knowledge and experiences' (1987: 325). On the basis of the map of reflective writing, they move through the reflective thinking process. Grumbacher suggests that other students can 'learn the process good problem solvers follow by practicing the process in logs or journals' (1987: 326).

From her reflections on how journals help physics students, Grumbacher also suggests that journals encourage students to initiate questions, and that once they have posed a question, they are inclined to work in order to answer them. She considers that journals help to provide the opportunity for students to 'play with the ideas of physics' in order better to understand.

Another form of journal in science subjects is the report. We described the research of McCrindle and Christensen (1995) on report writing in **biology** in Chapter 2. The research was focused more on the learning from the journals than on the quality of communication, but it could well be argued that the greater understanding and metacognitive ability that were achieved by the journal writing group are likely to contribute to the quality of reports.

Observation is relevant to report writing in science. Fulwiler (1986) describes how journal writing 'teaches people to see better.... I begin to look at the world differently because I know I will write about it because writing about anything causes me to notice it more fully'. He describes a use of a 'notebook' in **biology** in which students are asked not only to record what they see but also what they think about what they see. Writing informally, he suggests, they see better and better understand what they see.

English and allied subjects

There are many ways of using journals in the subject areas that make up English and drama. Several utilize the freer forms of self-expression as a means of improving other writing. Flynn (1986) used journals in **English** alongside a text as a means of increasing students' understanding of the text. The response to a literary text shifts from 'expression to transaction, from reader orientated to writer orientated' (1986: 209). Students were asked to write their personal responses to a particular text in journals and then to write a first draft of their account of the text. Flynn describes the first draft typically as too involved in the text and unfocused. In the final draft, the reader learns to view the text from a greater distance, seeing details that he or she has previously missed. Flynn argues that it is important for time to be spent in the exploratory phase, with written products being the result of an 'extended process of discovery' (1986: 213). She says 'pedagogical structures which encourage students to read and to write in stages also encourage them to transform their perceptions of texts which, in turn, may encourage them to transform their perceptions of their worlds and of themselves' (1986: 213).

Lindberg (1987) applies the use of journals in a manner different from that of Flynn to achieve a similar objective – of helping learners to gain a deeper understanding of texts. He uses a dialectical – or double entry – journal (see Chapter 3). Students write their observations of and reactions to the text on one side of the page. These may include 'times when your reading changes you are surprised or puzzled … something just does not fit … your first impression of the ending'. When the story is read, they are asked to go back and make sense of the observations. These journals are discussed in a planned series of 'conferences' (Chapter 8).

Gatlin (1987), again working with literary texts, started out with the anticipation of successful deep learning from journal work but reports how he failed to persuade his students to work comfortably and independently in journals. The situation, however, reversed when he began to share his own journal writings with his class. 'The result was dramatic because the rest of the class not only experienced a real example of a journal entry but they began to regard me as a fellow learner, not just an authority figure. This broke some thick ice in the class and brought about a real improvement in their journals and in our class discussions' (1987: 112).

Tama and Peterson (1991) use literary texts for a different, almost opposite, purpose to those above. While journals in the paragraphs above facilitate learning about the text and literature, these writers describe the use of journals in mediating learning about self from the reading of literature. Tama and Peterson select a group of texts around a theme such as the character of teachers – and through reading and reflecting in journals, students learn – or 'weigh and consider' as they quote from Francis Bacon – how it is to be a teacher.

Learning about a role is carried to a greater extreme in the example of journal use given by Craig from an example in **drama** (Dillon, 1983). Sister Craig describes how children (in this case) learned to become more secure in their roles in a drama production by writing a daily journal in role.

We have described how Lindberg used double entry journals to help students to understand meaning in a literary text. Joyce (www) uses a similar format in **information skills** classes to help students to evaluate sources of information. The page is divided into two. The students are asked to read an article or a chapter of a book, to read some quotations and to summarize or to respond to the material on one side of the journal. On the other side, they evaluate the material in terms of authenticity, currency, bias or overt point of view, reliability and so on. The journal entries support a discussion and students are asked to write up their discussion in their journals.

Kent (1987) lays a few ground-rules to guide students on use of journals in an introduction to **philosophy** course. In 'free writing', they are told to write what they like, but they must present the views of the subject accurately and logically. They are required to support any judgements they might make about the views. Kent suggests that the success of journals in his large class is that they exploit formal academic writing and informal self-expressive writing – and that for a subject like philosophy it is necessary to function in both.

The humanities and social sciences

Wagenaar introduced a journal in **sociology** in order to encourage students to relate the theory taught on the course to their own observations and experiences for the purposes of meeting 'the higher level cognitive objectives in her or his course'. (Wagenaar, 1984). He describes it as 'an intellectual exercise in reflexivity' which exploits the functions of evaluation and application (Bloom, 1956). Students were not asked to write about their feelings but from the examples given, feelings were present and acceptable in their expressions. The process of journal writing was relatively simple. Two elements were to be present in the journal – the observation of behaviour and the discussion in theoretical terms. There were two formats in which the students could write. They could either describe the observation and then relate it to theory – or they could combine the two. Wagenaar suggests that there are a number of areas of sociology where journal writing of this kind is helpful, and he cites Jensen (1979) who asked students to focus on one topic in the area of social problems in their journals for a term. The narrowing of the subject matter allows a wider range of consideration. For example, students could follow the topic in professional journals as well as in the popular press.

Steffens (1987) advocates the use of journals in **history** classes for a similar purpose to Wagenaar. He wishes the journal entries to provide a link between experiences and existing knowledge and the history topic in hand. In discussing the role of writing in history, he points out that history does not exist without writing '... doing history means writing history' (1987: 219). He acknowledges the importance of writing as communication but suggests that there is a further role, not as frequently exploited. Writing informally 'provides an opportunity to develop ideas, to "see" those ideas and to decide whether they disagree or agree with themselves.... We know a great deal more history than we can usually recall immediately' (1987: 219). He suggests that exploratory writing provides time and space for students to relate theory and new knowledge to what they discover that they know already.

In this form of journal, students were asked to write entries on a given topic in class and at home, interrelating the inputs and providing a personal response in the form of questions, speculation and doubts. Questions and tasks were used to generate 10 minutes of writing at the beginning of a class. To illustrate their diversity, some examples of the questions/tasks for the topic European Cultural History, 1880–1930 are:

> 'Vienna of the 1890s has been stigmatized as the training ground of Adolph Hitler. Was Paris of the 1890s any different?'
> 'What is the most interesting thing I have come to so far in my research paper?' (The research was a required task)
> 'List all the things for which Einstein is famous.'

Steffens also describes the use of journal entries to draw conclusions at the end of a class.

Brodsky and Meagher (1987) use a similar approach to journals in **political science**. One of the features of the teaching strategy was to ask students to complete some entries on assigned tasks and a given number of entries on subject matter of their choice. Evaluations of learning taking place in classes were also included. The journals were used as a means of initiating classroom discussion. Baltensperger (1987), working with **geography** students, describes a similar element in his work with classroom journals. He posed a question to students and asked them to write their responses first. He would then ask the question again, requesting oral reports based on the written ideas, and then would open the discussion for more general comment. He found this a valuable means of combating problems of poor response to oral questions posed in class.

There are a number of reports on journals in **psychology** in the literature, with those by Hettich probably the best known. In two papers, separated by 14 years, Hettich advocated similar functions for journals in psychology – similar as well to the purposes advocated by Wagenaar (above) (Hettich, 1976, 1990). Journals were seen to help students to connect course learning to their real experiences and observations. The emphasis is on the course material, and instructions indicated that entries could contain 'examples that show comprehension of the concept; application or experimentation with principles; and analysis, evaluation and synthesis of course concepts' (Hettich, 1990).

Journals were used in a different manner in a course in adolescent psychology (McManus, 1986). While they still served to relate theory to practice, an important part of the students' learning in practice focused on a series of regular meetings of the college students with local adolescents. The journals charted the learning from the experience of the meetings. Another example of journal use in psychology is most unusual. Terry (1984) asked students to record instances of forgetting during the period of the course on memory. They were required to write the situation, the activities in which they were engaged and their emotional state and to consider the factors involved in forgetting and retrieval.

In a project to investigate the impact of different forms of writing in **anthropology**, Creme (1998) describes three different forms of journals in a social anthropology department. Project logs accompanied a first-year course that introduced the theoretical and conceptual basis to anthropology research. The logs were used in a research project and contained recordings and reflection on the records. The second form is called a record of study. Students developed an account of their learning from different sources throughout the course with a focus on the development of 'understanding of central course concepts'. The third form of journal was used in a first-year multidisciplinary course on death. In their journals, students explored their reactions to various accounts of death and to their personal experiences.

Languages

Mülhaus and Löschmann (1997) discuss issues relating to **foreign language learning** in modularized higher education. The change from integrated programmes to the accumulation of modules means that students enrolling on a module are likely to have diverse backgrounds in relation to the subject matter. A distance learning approach was adopted with students using workshop time for advice and progress checks. With this approach, the writers considered that students needed to give attention to their learning strategies and they used journals to address that need. Journals included the written work of students – video summaries, vocabulary lists, worksheet tasks and self-reflective comments. A marking scheme assessed 'the interaction with the material and the depth of the learning process as evident from the students' vocabulary lists, translations and comments' (1997: 25). The comments on learning made in the journals both formed the basis of workshops and were shared for others to try.

There are aspects in common between the approach above and that of Finch (www). Finch used journals with 'false beginners' – Korean students needing language skills to cope both with learning in English and needing new skills and confidence to cope with the cultural differences in learning. Finch's journal was very structured, with questionnaires for completion about skills and attitudes in language learning, self-evaluation forms and a blank section for personal reflections.

Arts subjects

The first three examples in this section on journals in **arts subjects** may look the same, but they have different purposes. One form of journal that is a natural accompaniment to the creation of music and drama is the project type of journal where the development of ideas is recorded and considered reflectively in the journal. The aim is to enhance the thought processes that contribute to the project. With **art and design** students, Davies (1998) set a similar journal that accompanies project work, but where the main aim is one of assessment. He suggests that there can be too much focus on the outcome of art student work and not on the all-important process of it. The journals demonstrate process, and assessment is on this basis. A third example of journal that may coincide with those above is a journal that itself generates creative ideas. Rainer's (1978) many ideas for types of journal include the development of what she calls 'a sourcebook for creative projects'.

The fourth example in this section is different. Ambrose (1987) describes a **music** journal. Like many others, initially the journal was a means of improving writing. Students were asked to write their comments about concerts attended, music heard and books read about music. However, the journals served the purpose of monitoring the students' listening behaviour. They were expected, for example, to attend a certain number of concerts. Ambrose observed that the written work of students improved.

Business and law

Business subjects range from number-based to literary studies. November (1993) makes a comment about his subject, **commerce,** that may apply quite widely in this range of subjects. He suggests that the study environment is not always conducive to deep approaches to learning (Chapter 2). He used journals in order to deepen the quality of learning in a final-year course. Over the time that he used this method, he found that the best results occurred when considerable guidance on the journal writing was given. One method that he reports is to ask students to write an 'agenda' – a list of problems or issues of concern, and then to examine each in a systematic manner. Every so often he asked students to review the kinds of questions that are raised in their writing.

Both Wolf (1980) and Ficher (1990), using journals for **administration** and **marketing** studies respectively, indicate that an important purpose of the method is the provision of a means of linking the classroom learning with the business world. Wolf's instructions to students were to focus on a 'moment or event' from four perspectives. The first is outer experience (as a third-person description), the next is one of reflection and generalization to deepen understanding, the third stage is 'inner experience' – a subjective account. The fourth is more reflection and generalization to connect the current focus with previous experiences. There is an 'appendix' which represents a periodic overview of themes and agendas for future learning. This work was based on the Kolb cycle (Kolb, 1984 – described in Chapter 2).

Ficher's students were asked to make one journal entry per class, relating 'real world' observations to the class material, using the correct terminology. The recognition of this relationship was the first purpose which journals were to fulfil. Another was to 'increase student sensitivity to consumer behaviour', a third was to increase participation in the class and the fourth was to improve oral and written communication skills.

Elkins (1985) describes the use of journals in the context of **law**. The journals were a means of counteracting the uncaring and subject-centred attitudes that he describes in legal education. In the journals 'legal education is presented… as it is personally experienced, as individual students "see" it, "feel" it, and make it part of their lives'.

Perhaps the idea that journals contribute in any subject to 'making it part' of the student's life is a reminder that most of the applications of journals in the different subjects that are mentioned above apply far more broadly. With a bit of thought they can facilitate learning in different ways in many contexts.

Chapter 5

Journals in professional education and development

Introduction

This chapter concerns the use of journals in professional education and professional development. Most examples of journals that are described in the literature are in the initial phase of professional education, but there is increasing use of reflective writing in portfolios at practising professional stages, often in the form of a professional portfolio. In order to provide an overview of journals in professional education and development, the chapter is divided into four sections. The first concerns journals that are orientated towards the development of the self as a professional. The second section concerns journals that improve practice, often by making the link between theory and practice. The next section concerns journals that focus on professional empowerment by raising and working with socio-political awareness. Lastly there is a section which reviews examples of the ways in which journals can support elements of educational programmes. As we have said before, however, most journals are set for or fulfil several purposes and that is the case with many journals in this chapter. We have not made a division between practising professionals and novices. In this age of lifelong learning there is a sense that education and development are continuous – only the content and methods may vary.

The previous chapter reviewed many uses of journals in academic disciplines. It is difficult to draw a line between non-vocational and professional education as there are elements of professional education that are subject orientated and aspects of subject-orientated learning that are common to professional development learning. Engineering students become engineers as much as education students become teachers and yet the former tend to be seen as less vocational than the latter.

Journals seem to be most prevalent in nursing and education. In my book on reflection, I speculated as to why reflection seemed to be so much a part of the ethos of these professions. For example, both have tended to be more commonly taken up by women who are more reflective by nature (Clarke, James and Kelly, 1996). Both professions rely on interpretive knowledge which is socially constructed and not rooted in a body of 'fact' (Schön, 1987). Both also rely on decisions made 'on the spot' with unpredictable situations being relatively common. Action is what counts but the consequences of action can be critical.

We have said above that journals in professional education and development are described here in four sections. We have not dealt with professions separately – it seems fruitful that ideas should flow across professions – though some differences are noticeable. Teacher education students, for example, are commonly asked to consider their own experiences of education, schools, teachers and so on. In general, the journals of nurses seem to be more orientated towards the nature of their practice. It is worth noting that journals in professional education and development seem to have exploited more often retrospective and anticipatory considerations – they flow backwards over the past, or forwards, preparing for the future.

Journals in the development of self as a professional

We have commented before on the notion that professional development involves self-development. This is more likely to be particularly the case in professions where the nature of activity demands a response from the whole person. To facilitate learning or to nurture educational development involves the whole person – cognitively and emotionally – and a similar scenario is true of the art of patient care. Because most journal writing draws expression or exploration of emotion and attitude into the 'open' in writing, it has the potential to link personal and professional education and development. Additionally, with emotions and attitudes expressed, there is an unusually good possibility of examination and modification. Where they can remain hidden, the opportunity for change is limited.

In the context of the development of self as a professional, a number of writers talk of the development of 'voice'. Oberg and Underwood (1992) wrote a joint paper in which they describe the dialogue journal between them, one as teacher educator and one as student (Underwood). The accounts describe Underwood finding her 'inner voice', her 'own tale in the telling'. In this process, she recognized herself as 'becoming … whole, both the creator and interpreter of meaning'. Canning (1991), however, notes the later reflections of qualified teachers who also felt that they were finding a 'voice' in their reflective processes. They suggested that the potential 'voice' of students is often subdued by their training 'to please, to defer to professors and supervisors for good grades and positive evaluations'. Others of Canning's group felt that their voices were thwarted by mechanistic attitudes to the teaching process by administrators. One of her subjects rationalized: 'I may not be able to change decisions … but now I know what I'm thinking.'

Wolf (1989) illustrates the use of the metaphor of voice in journals in the education of gerontologists. Her aim was to counteract the tendency of the literature and theory of ageing to 'objectify' and distance the ageing process. Her concern is that students will consider that older people are 'out there' rather than a part of themselves. She talks about the focus that the journal gives to encouraging students to hear the inner voice, to 'open up', to articulate the fears of ageing. She says: 'In learning to articulate our inner voice, we must focus on ourselves; the act of composing our thoughts in journal form helps shape this activity.'

It is interesting to observe that while most of the teacher education papers on the use of journals concern self-development in relation to the work role, similar papers written in the caring professions often focus on the relationship of the novice professional in relationship to her clients. As with Wolf, above, Landeen, Byrne and Brown (1992) are concerned with the role of journals in developing appropriate attitudes of students of psychiatric nursing to their patients. In an experimental study, one group of students kept journals in which they had to describe the most significant event of each day in their clinical setting. They were then to 'reflect on the impact that event had for them in terms of understanding a client situation, their own attitudes in the situation and future learning needs as a result of the event'. There were two control groups. The findings suggested that journal writing was a positive aid to students in exploration and change of their attitudes. They were able to become more comfortable in working with these patients apparently as a result of the journal work.

Strengthening 'voice' and increasing comfort in professional situations are among a mass of qualities that are related to journal writing – which amount, in general terms, to increasing confidence in the professional role. Ashbury, Fletcher and Birtwhistle (1993) used journals in a communications course with first-year students in medicine. Here the emphases were on the development of confident communications with potential patients, personal reflection and evaluation of the course experience. Ashbury et al comment that the students' journals enabled them to become aware:

> of many of the concerns and struggles of medical students as they progressed through first year issues…. (The) students identified and addressed issues related to their future role as doctors, their suitability for that career, the effect of their gender on that role, patients' perceptions of doctors, … and the complexities of communication, interviewing and learning in small groups.
>
> (Ashbury et al, 1996)

Among others reporting on this development of confidence are (for teaching students) Dart et al (1998), Rovegno (1992) and for nurses Dimino (1988).

Another type of journal focuses more deliberately on the progression through and recording of the experiences of developing professionals. What is termed 'journal' here might there be called by such terms as portfolio, a professional profile or record of achievement (James and Denley, 1993). Such documents may play a large part in the assessment of the course or may be used to assess the professional for probationary periods or for promotion. The reflective writing element in them may be less important as a means of learning, and more important as a means of linking the elements of the portfolio into a more coherent presentation (Paulson, Paulson and Meyer, 1991). It is worth noting that, while the examples we have given above are developed concurrently with the accumulation of the experiences, a portfolio may be developed from past recorded experiences, as in the case of the accreditation of prior learning or PhDs by presentation of a portfolio of work. While these are accompanied by reflective writing, they begin to slide outside our definition of journals. The reflective writing is more of a summarizing account and is not necessarily progressive. It may, however, be a powerful source of learning, allowing the writers to see previous elements of their work in a different light that has inferences for future activity.

It is somewhat in this way that autobiography has a role alongside or incorporated within journal writing. Autobiography is also retrospective, but elements of autobiography writing are often a part or an exercise in journal writing (Knowles, 1993). The major use of autobiography is in teacher education. The assumption is that during childhood contacts with learning, school and teachers, a range of emotions, attitudes, understandings and personal beliefs develop about the educational situation. Along the lines of constructivist thinking, these 'personal theories'(Griffiths and Tann, 1992), represented in the cognitive structure of students (Chapter 2), form the basis for professional learning. The elements of prior learning are likely to be represented as 'knowledge-in-pieces' – a relatively incoherent foundation on which to build a future teacher's orientation to his or her profession (Winitzky and Kauchak, 1997). Making this knowledge, emotion and attitude explicit allows it to be examined and related constructively to new learning. A journal is an ideal vehicle for this exercise since it can provide present and anticipated future contexts alongside the working in the past and it can provide the opportunities to return to the past experiences on many different occasions.

Personal experiences of autobiography journal exercises suggest that the context of the present is influential on the nature of memories that emerge on any particular occasion. To take account of this phenomenon, Grumet (1987) recommends the use of the *currere* technique (after Pinar, 1975) in which the past, present and future anticipations of an experience are considered at the same time (see Chapter 10). An illustration of the use of autobiography, present and future considerations is provided by Aspinwall (1986). Interestingly this paper is based on work with a practising teacher, not a student teacher. It is worthy of note that there do not appear to be reports of the use of autobiography in the health care professions where personal experiences and perceptions of illness and health care would seem to be equally relevant to professional education and development.

In a later paper, Grumet develops her views on autobiography in teacher education. She suggests that it is not just the writing part of the process that is important, but the reading of the accounts as well. She says:

> Reading autobiography invites its reader to discriminate the particular from the general in her own account. It makes it possible to ground an approach to pedagogy in what she has known and experienced without requiring her to impose her experience on the students. It invites the individual to attend to the differences as well as to the similarities between the world in which she came to form and the worlds that her students come from.
>
> (Grumet, 1989)

Grumet goes on to suggest that a further stage of working with autobiography can be the critical consideration of the material from the perspectives of educational philosophy, psychology, sociology and history. She sees this process as linking the realm of private thought to that of public knowledge so that the validity of personal thought processes is recognized and becomes a part of professional education and development.

Journals in the development of practice

Perhaps the most common use of journals in professional education is in the context of practice or in moving between classroom theory and situations of practice. This is a process that is superficially similar to that described in the previous chapter where students made better sense of their theory by linking it to common events in 'the real world' (eg Hettich, 1990). However, in the professional context the emphasis is not always on the development of more sound theory, but more often on the enhancement of practice. This is particularly relevant in the face of political pressure to make – in particular, teacher training – more practical (Griffiths and Tann, 1992).

Dart *et al* (1998) studied the way in which graduate trainee teachers used their journals as a means of relating theory to practice. In the early part of their one-year course, students would comment on theory and not relate it to practice situations ('no connection'). At a later stage a second form of link between theory and practice emerged. Here theory was used to inform practice and generally the reverse of this did not occur at that time. The examples of student journal comments suggest that students were demonstrating this in practical situations or in metacognitive comments about their own learning. An example of the former is of a student who recognized that a teacher is not 'a provider of knowledge' but a 'facilitator of learning' – and then goes on to suggest to herself ways of facilitating learning such as 'make things relevant and enjoyable'. An example of the latter is where a student comments on how her use of concept maps was helpful to her methods of learning. Later still in the course, Dart *et al* observed some journal entries that demonstrate both theory to practice and practice to theory links.

Journals have also been used to support what is called reflective practice – both in its development and in its function. However, there is a difficulty in generalizing in these areas because reflective practice has different meanings and connotations. In an interesting metaphor, Wellington (1991) described the qualities of reflective practice as those of a 'tenacious' city wild flower which 'vibrates with vitality, raising our awareness and calling us from passivity into action'. In somewhat less colourful language, my earlier work on reflection (Moon, 1999a) suggests that reflective practice has been used to describe a set of abilities and skills, to indicate the taking of a critical stance (see next section in this chapter), an orientation to problem solving or a state of mind. Journals have a role in the development of all of these capacities and attitudes, as the following comments and examples will indicate.

The instructions for journal writing for reflective practice vary. In some examples of the use of journals, the instruction has been to reflect freely, and in others, structure is imposed in a variety of manners. In an example of the former, Hoover (1994) describes the journals of two teaching students. One made satisfactory use of the journal to make sense of his practical experiences. The other, however, increasingly used her journal to work out her 'identity crisis' with regard to teaching and she eventually left the programme. It is a moot point as to whether the journal performed a useful task for the latter student. Hoover indicates that she did not see this as a successful use of journal activities and that more structure could have guided writing into 'deliberations about educational principles and practice'.

In a relatively simple example of structure in journals used to generate reflective practice, Sparkes-Langer *et al* (1990) describe a journal assignment in which they asked students each day to describe one successful and one less successful event of the day. They were asked to consider the context and issues raised, and focus on 'why' questions about the events. Another relatively simple structure was given as an option by Francis (1995). Teaching students were asked initially to describe an event ('a brief summary of the key points'), to indicate new insights that came out of the session, then to consider emerging questions and to provide a personal reaction. Against the map of reflective writing in Chapter 2, this guidance might seem to skip the act of reflection itself.

In keeping with the map of reflective writing, Morrison (1996) is concerned that teaching students 'move on' in their thinking through journals. He bases his work with journals and other means of encouraging reflective practice on two models. In the first model, the reflection is directed towards the actions of the student. It uses Schön's (1983) notions of 'reflection-in-action' and 'reflection-on-action', and poses questions to help students in their reflection. Students are asked, for example, to consider their personal, professional, academic and evaluative development in such areas as increasing knowledge, attitudinal changes and 'the expansion (in depth and breadth) of their vision'. In the second part of the model, reflection is seen more in terms of empowerment and political awareness. Such considerations, as we have suggested earlier, have the potential to deepen reflective activity. Issues concerning the functioning of the self in a particular setting (Prawat, 1991) are related to the experiences of the students in their strands of development.

In the field of nursing, Johns (1994) also provides a list of questions that can guide the learning from experience. Like Morrison, the first questions encourage the description of the experience. The next section is headed 'Reflection'. In it he proposes questions such as 'What was I trying to achieve?', 'What were the consequences of my action for myself, the patient/family, the people I work with?' and three further questions about the feelings of 'myself', the patient, and 'How do I know how the patient felt about it?'. He brings in 'Influencing factors' of a personal (internal) nature and external nature and queries what sources of knowledge 'did/should have influenced my decision-making?'. It is interesting to note that this set of questions concerning influencing factors, which would come under 'additional information' in the map of reflective writing, follow what Johns calls 'reflection'. In the map the additional information is brought into the reflective process.

The last questions that Johns recommends concern the learning that emerges from the process of reflection – any changes in feelings, proposed changes in behaviour or understanding of wider issues (eg ethics).

Heath's (1998) work is also in the field of nursing and, as we have indicated earlier, she proposes the use of double entry journals (see Chapter 3). A valuable aspect of her use of journals is the recognition of the need for different forms of guidance for those more advanced in the profession or more able at reflective writing. The general pattern of this progression is from the simplest form of reflection in which the practitioner realizes that practice is an important source of learning and knowledge. At the next stage there is recognition that the learning has implications for future practice and there is some linking of theory and practice. At the most advanced stage, there is a broadening and deepening of the content of reflection.

Structured journals support practice and help a student to make sense of the experiences; however, in these new and challenging situations the free-writing areas of journals can act with all the qualities of purely personal journals. They can act as 'friend', somewhere to vent feelings, to note new enthusiasms or to sort out the daily new dilemmas and difficulties.

Journals used to develop socio-political awareness

We have mentioned above a few writers who have included socio-political or ethical reasoning in journal tasks and we commented that dealing with these issues can be an effective manner of deepening the reflection process. A few other writers, however, have focused directly on the development of critical awareness of this kind. Sparkes-Langer and Colton (1991) distinguish the development of critique by suggesting that cognitive elements of reflection 'emphasize how teachers make decisions', but 'the critical approach stresses the substance that drives the thinking – the experiences, beliefs, sociopolitical values and goals...'. Proponents of this approach have been, for example, Smyth (1987) and Tripp (1987). Smyth observes the 'skills-related way in which most in-service education had been conceived and enacted'. He sees work of this sort on teacher improvement as 'intellectually bankrupt'. He considers that what is important is to 'challenge the myth that somehow classroom teaching is, or should be, a detached, neutral ... and value-free activity'. The work on which Smyth based this was with a group of teachers involved in 'active critique and an uncovering of the tensions that exist between particular teaching practices and the larger cultural and social contexts in which teaching is embedded'. By working in a group, and using journals to record classroom incidents, they sought to move beyond the technical interpretations of the social settings of classrooms as representing the source of limitations on teaching. They re-evaluated these sources of limitation as elements in a system in which any 'rules, roles and structures' could potentially be challenged.

A description of the incidents was the first of four stages in developing the critique. The second stage questioned first the meaning behind the teaching ('informing'). This involved seeking theories that lay behind the description of the event or relationships between elements in it. The 'reconstructing' phase concerned the manner in which the event might have been handled differently, and the 'confronting' phase considers the assumptions, beliefs and values that underlie events, the manner in which they are maintained, and whose interest they serve.

Smyth's work was undertaken with practising teachers; however, the principles of it are applied in teacher education. There is some question as to whether student teachers are sufficiently knowledgeable to challenge the system into which they move (Moon, 1999a).

Using journals to support elements of educational programmes

There are a number of examples of journal use that support the particular content of educational programmes. One involves problem-based learning in dentistry (Wetherell and Mullins, 1996). Problem-based learning (PBL) is becoming increasingly common in dentistry, apparently following the example set in medical schools. In this case, journals are used in two areas of a programme to: 'formalize reflection, (provide) an outlet for personal feeling; an opportunity for feedback about a student's progress and about the course; ... a summary of the year's work; and a means whereby students and teachers gain insight into the learning process'.

One use of journals by Wetherell and Mullins is in an oral diagnosis course, in the setting of a pain clinic. The course was intended to increase students' responsibility for their learning and self-development. The journal was a vehicle for expression of feelings and to communicate issues of concern to their tutors. Students were asked to write about anxieties and ways in which they felt they could gain more from the clinic experience. The journal content was discussed in one-to-one tutorials. After modifications, around three-quarters of the students favoured the method. Among specific reasons for this, the journal's provision of a record of cases and its value as a 'checklist of things to be learned or done' were cited in particular.

Wetherell and Mullins also report on journals used in their first year (PBL) dentistry courses. Students faced four 'streams' and a variety of unfamiliar forms of input. They were given a general introduction to journals as a tool for learning with discussion and a demonstration of existing journals. Their writing covered material from the four streams and they were encouraged to explore personal reactions to their experiences. As in many other examples of journal work, this provided staff with valuable feedback on the curriculum. The journals were read and helpful comments were made, but there was no graded assessment.

In the context of problem-based learning, it is interesting to note comment by Yinger and Clark (1981) about their uses of journals with teachers. '... given the opportunity to write about and reflect on what they were doing, remarkable and exciting changes took place. Much to their surprise, they found themselves solving problems ... that had previously been wearing them down.'

Chapter 6

Learning journals and personal development

Introduction

There are no sharp lines to be drawn between personal and professional development and we have said that it is doubtful that one can develop as an adequate professional in the broader sense without parallel personal developments. The idea of personal development in learning journals, however, generates a wealth of approaches and styles. Many of the approaches to journals that are included in this chapter can be or are applied to enrich journal writing in professional and formal education learning. Perhaps, too, the more formal approaches of journals in education can help to focus the personal development journal styles towards outcomes of learning rather than descriptive accounts.

The structure of the chapters of this book so far has more or less spelt itself out during the phase of literature review. However, this is not the case with the material on personal development journals. Such is the range of enthusiastic writing about personal journals that it proves difficult to determine a structure within which to make a worthwhile account which, as well as being informative, captures the rich potential of this form of writing. After several perusals of the literature on personal development journals, some headings that roughly covered the field reluctantly emerged and now form the basis of the chapter.

Some general issues in the writing of personal learning journals

The intention to engage in personal journal writing is almost certainly far more prevalent than is the practice. It might be interesting to muse on what all the purchasers of blank journal pages have in their minds. The purchases are most common at new year and it is likely, for that reason, that the often flat after-Christmas days of early January are those most commonly recorded before the habit tails off. Another start-time for journals is on holiday or travelling somewhere. It was interesting to observe, recently, the sale of blank books labelled 'journal' at airports.

While we take in the full range of journal writing that is not work-related in this chapter, the focus is largely on journals that are written for longer than the first day of a holiday, and with more purpose than description of events. The focus is on situations where there is intention to 'move on' personally. The ways of 'moving on' represent the headings of this chapter but as in previous situations in this book, there are overlaps, and original intentions may yield different outcomes. Personal development journals may be for 'moving on' by way of:

- provision of personal support;
- establishment of personal identity;
- therapy;
- exploration, widening of experience or awareness;
- self-organization;
- support of creativity;
- the development or support of spirituality.

Because this chapter involves the notion of self-development, it is worth dwelling on what this term might mean because it is relevant to the manner in which some journals are used. When applying the notion of reflection in personal development contexts in my previous book (Moon, 1999a), I suggested that personal development could usefully be seen as functioning in a deficit or non-deficit situation. The former represents situations of counselling or therapy where the aim is to reach a perceived state of normality. The latter represents 'growth' or the aim to reach a more successful state. Based on Eraut's (1994) work, it was convenient to see personal development as operating in three notional stages – of self-awareness, self-improvement and self-empowerment – the effort to be aware, the effort to go beyond this and improve, and the reaching out for forms of emancipation.

Journals for personal support

'Personal support' is a term to cover a range of ideas around what are probably the most usual reasons for using personal journals – for finding direction, for understanding the self, for keeping things in balance. A journal is a place in which the writers can be authentically themselves and can weave their way through the portrayed selves that are seen by others. Bruner's (1990) concept of 'the construction of a longitudinal version of self' seems particularly relevant to journal writing.

Some have described their journals as a friend or as company, for example, through transitions. Bridges (1980) suggests that a journal can be particularly helpful during experiences such as divorce or career change – particularly in the space between endings and beginnings that he calls the 'neutral zone'. Journals can provide the personal space within which to undertake 'rites of passage'. Somewhat allied to the notion of 'friend' is the notion of nurturance. Cooper (1991) suggests that 'Writing in a journal is … a way to attend to the self, to care for and to feed oneself'. Bruce (www) refers to the work of clinical psychologists that has 'proven that writing (in journals) contributes directly to … physical health'. He talks about a drop in visits to physicians, fewer days' absence from work and improved general health.

In elaboration of this, Cooper goes on to talk about journals also as a place for 'dumping anger, guilt or fear instead of dumping it on those we love' (1991: 105). Rainer (1978) talks of 'putting a scream in the diary'. From personal experience, helpful 'screams' may come in the form of letters written large or with a heavy pen, or written across the page. Working on catharsis in Progoff's (1975) Intensive Journal or with Rainer's techniques might be a matter, for example, of writing a dialogue (Chapter 10) with the agency that represents the cause of the anger – be it person or organization (etc).

Some journal writing appeals to a strength or wisdom that can be availed through the act of writing reflectively. For example, Rainer talks of the 'silver-lining voice' that comes into her writing, giving her advice, and in a somewhat different example Fox (1982) refers to the support that journal writing gave to a client of his in his attempts to give up smoking. Progoff formalizes the notion of guidance from wisdom in one of the sections of the Intensive Journal in which writers dialogue in imagination with a person or being who has been a source of wisdom in their lives.

Writing a journal over a period of time provides personal support also in the perspective on personal attitudes and behaviour that it provides. From personal experience, one of the most useful sections of the Intensive Journal is the 'period log'. The period log is a section for review of a period of life in which there has been a common theme or direction. More than most other journal writing activities, it provides a sense of perspective, a sense of rhythm and change and sometimes a repeat of themes in life. It generates a sense of balance in which it is easier to place the peaks and troughs – the 'mountains and molehills' (Rainer, 1978).

Journals for establishing personal identity

The lives of some people are obviously rich. Before the end of their teens they have undergone more socially valued experiences than others ever experience. To gather self-esteem enough to rise beyond an impoverished lifestyle can be difficult for many without these socially valued experiences. Progoff's journal was part of a programme for a group of unemployed New York people who were training to take on work as nurse's aides, security guards and other such jobs (Kaiser, 1981). Most were new immigrants, were black and had few opportunities to help themselves. Ninety per cent of them were keeping the journal after six months, and most succeeded in maintaining the posts or bettering themselves. The programme officials attributed much of the success of the programme to the use of the journal and the manner in which it brought them into touch with their inner selves.

Along the same lines, Hallberg (1987) talks of journals being 'person-making'. He suggests that the use of journals (such as that of Progoff) 'is far more powerful and far-reaching in its effects than is generally recognized. [It is] ... working to change that student's enduring attitudes, values and sense of personal identity' (1987: 289).

Becoming aware of the range of experiences and valuing them builds a sense of identity or personhood. Fox (1982) describes how a client in therapy, a 14-year-old who had been in foster care for most of his life, gathered 'fragments of his life' – photos, ticket stubs and so on – in order to 'define himself' and begin to build a self-image. A journal of this sort serves to position an individual in the present, with an understood past and a clearer future. Rainer (1978) talks of 'rereading yourself' by reading through journal entries. She says: 'the diarist comes to see patterns of experience and personality.... The patterns are completely individual and deepen the understanding of one's own nature' (1978: 265). Similarly, Cooper (1991) talks of journals as 'a way to tell our own story, a way to learn who we have been, who we are and who we are becoming. We literally become teachers and researchers in our own lives, empowering ourselves in the process' (1991: 98). Empowerment is seen as the 'integration of ... own needs, values and desires with the often conflicting views of society or the workplace' (Cooper, 1991: 108).

Journals in therapy

Clearly, in considering journals in therapy, there is an overlap with the previous section. However, not all uses of journals in therapy are associated with the establishment of personal identity. In a further example, Fox describes the use of journal writing to support behaviour changes and shifts in attitude. One client, for example, found it helpful to examine his smoking behaviour in detail and to locate the type of anxiety that was relieved through smoking. He managed subsequently to give up smoking. Another client, with very rigid attitudes and behaviour, took on a more relaxed personality through writing a journal. His subject matter initially was formal, but he progressed through free writing and 'rambling' and was able to 'turn away from logical, sequentially ordered thinking towards freer contact with experience and feeling'.

Another therapeutic use of journal writing is rehearsal of future events that evoke fear. By writing about the (future) event, imagining going through it and behaving calmly, and rereading/reliving the material several times, there is likely to be a beneficial effect on behaviour at the time of the event itself. An example of this application might be a driving test. Rainer (1978) describes behaviour rehearsal in a considerably less clinical context of engendering eroticism, where she suggests that the writer should practise in her journal making requests for fulfilment of her sexual desires.

It was in a context of psychotherapy that Progoff developed the structure of the Intensive Journal. He would ask clients to write in a loose-leaf notebook to record the events of their inner lives. Through noticing the pattern of questions that he asked of clients in relation to their writing, be began to formulate the sections that were subsequently the structure of the published version (Progoff, 1975).

Journals for exploring, widening experience or awareness

A large range of journal writing belongs in this group. It includes the old idea of a commonplace book, which was like a scrapbook of everyday life. It probably includes most travel and holiday journals that are written to accompany the exploration of external physical journeys (Mallon, 1984). In this respect, Fulwiler's (1986) likening of journal entries to snapshots of life is helpful. He suggests that because he writes a journal and may write about what he experiences, he experiences it with greater awareness.

Journals may also accompany an internal mental journey. There are many descriptions of journals of internal mental journeys of exploration in the literature. Creme's (1998) example (Chapter 4) of death journals is one. Another is the sex journal undertaken by Anderson's (1982) students in the context of a psychology class. The students were asked to keep a journal of their 'observations of sex in the environment, magazines, TV, peoples' interactions etc. and [their] reactions to these observations'. Although the context of this exercise was academic, much of the learning that resulted seems to have been personal and over half of the students reported changing their behaviour or lifestyle as a result of the exercise. As they tried to make sense of what they recorded, they often gained insights. One said, 'As I write this, I realize how, for a lot of women, sex and fear are so interrelated. What do men fear? Women fear men.' Along similar lines, we referred above to Rainer's suggestion of the use of journals to explore eroticism and she also mentions the discovery of joy.

Rainer also suggests that the exploration of a range of personal problems can lead to their transformation. The outcome of an exploration may have significant effects. Knowing about personal capacities enables one better to appreciate the capacities in others, and thus to adapt one's behaviour towards others. It is as if the self is externalized for easier study. Similarly, in a professional development situation, we have previously mentioned Wolf's work with gerontology students who were asked to explore their attitudes towards age and ageing. In so doing, they confronted some difficult issues in themselves, such as acknowledgement of a fear of the old, and of old age (Wolf, 1989).

Sometimes the exploration of an issue in journals comes not from a direct confrontation with the object, but by treating it metaphorically. Metaphor can be a way of making explicit the personal theories by which we live (Griffiths and Tann, 1992). It may be a matter of applying metaphors to situations in order to make new understanding from them. For example, Cooper (1991) describes a situation in which a woman described herself as like a diaper pin in her family, 'holding the fabric of our lives together and keeping the crap cleaned off'. She says she is ready to pull out the pin: 'But must I hurt my family to pull out and let the fabric of the diaper find new shape and form – while I let the process of reshaping begin?'(1991: 102).

Joanna Field (Marion Milner) frequently used metaphor in her use of journals as a means of personal exploration of herself and her abilities to paint (Field, 1951; Milner, 1957, 1987). In her 1951 book, Field describes finding the method of free association as a means to uncovering the deeper meanings of her patterns of behaviour (see page 10).

In another book, written a little later, Milner (now using her own name, and a practising psychoanalyst) records, in a similar way, a further personal project of learning to paint (Milner, 1957). In 1987, she returned to the more generalized theme in *Eternity's Sunrise: A Way of Keeping a Diary* (Milner, 1987), now using metaphor as a means of structuring the manner in which she works in her diary. She focuses on the significance of the 'small private moments that came nuzzling into my thoughts, asking for attention' (synopsis). She interprets these 'bead memories' as 'bridges' or points of integration for the different aspects of mental functioning – feeling, reason and imagination, regarding them as having particular importance for the passage of her consciousness.

We began this section with reference to journals that accompany a journey, whether physical or mental. It is worth noting that Progoff's view of the metaphor of journey is different. He considers that there is a flow within our lives and when we begin to tap into it, we flow with it. Kaiser's (1981) interpretation is: 'There is an underground stream of images in all of us…. When we enter it, we ride where it wants to go.'

Journals for self-organization

To most people in professional or everyday life, a diary or sometimes even a journal means a small book in which to record events in the future as an *aide mémoire* and an aid to self-organization. One direction in which these have developed is in the 'pocket organizer' mode which was introduced a few years ago with specially punched paper to ensure that people were largely tied to purchasing expensive packs of paper. On the whole, this form of diary is a means of recording and noting, and not a journal in the sense of this book. Not very different from this idea, however, are means of working with journals that do facilitate the organization of one's life and which incorporate sections for the development of ideas. These do come into the range of this book. Most of what I write on this comes from my own experience but I see others using similar 'notebooks' or 'workbooks'. The word that seems most clearly to describe the way I use my book is 'thinkplace' because it is an aid to my thinking about work or life in progress. It is described as an example in Chapter 9.

Journals to support creativity

In one sense, all journal writing is creative. We construct meanings in the act of writing and creativity is part of the nature of reflective writing. We also need to acknowledge that specifically creative thoughts or insights can emerge unexpectedly from writing about anything. Sometimes the skill is in the recognition of the value of these thoughts. This section deals with journal work and writing that has a particular aim of generating creative ideas.

Sometimes a whole journal is devoted towards support or generation of creative ideas. Milner's (1957) description of learning to paint is a powerful example and it is both to its credit and its loss that it is so closely tied to psychoanalytical theory. Alternatively the search for creativity may be focused in journal activities. A number of activities with this function are described in the last chapter (Chapter 10). One that seems particularly relevant is the 'dialogue with works' (Progoff, 1975) in which a written dialogue is held with a proposed or ongoing project. It is a way of focusing on the intrinsic qualities of the project or 'work' and of avoiding the pressure of rationality or the influence of habit or others. Rainer (1978) includes a chapter on the use of journals to expand creativity in which she applies the various diary techniques.

There seem to be a number of ways in which journal writing might enhance creativity. Miller (1979) suggests that the act of writing may generate creative ideas but also that 'writing the immediate thoughts makes more "room" for new avenues of thinking…'. She suggests that writing allows the mind to 'explore more freely since we do not run the risk of losing our previous thoughts'. This may indicate why a project journal can come to feel so important (Chapter 9).

Working with dreams is a different means of generating ideas that are unexpected, but this inconveniently depends on the somewhat unpredictable process of dreaming and remembering dreams (Shohet, 1985). From personal experience, Progoff's techniques of reaching 'twilight' states are a more reliable means of accessing sources of 'the unexpected'. 'Twilight imagery' is a state in which one is deeply relaxed and has attention 'turned inwards'. Images begin to arise and they are recorded. The very act of recording and valuing the images seems to induce more images. Work in this mode 'feels' highly creative, but it may or may not have obvious application to any particular current issue. In a personal experience of such a session, what I subsequently called 'the bear-mouse' creature arose as an image. For a reason I cannot understand, it was a source of enormous joy on that day, and on later occasions whenever it arose in my mind. Its appearance brought feelings of great creativity and potential.

Writing a journal may also capture ideas for creative activities or as memories – like the notebook that is graphically described by Didion (1968):

> I sometimes delude myself about why I keep a notebook, imagine that some thrifty virtue derives from preserving everything observed. See enough and write it down, I tell myself, and then, some morning when the world seems drained of wonder… – on that bankrupt morning, I will simply open my notebook and there

it will all be, a forgotten account with accumulated interest, paid passage to the world out there.

(Didion, 1968: 115,116)

The development or support of spirituality

Journal writing can be an important activity in the development of both secular and religious spirituality. We have described in other chapters Walker's use of journals with potential leaders in a religious community (Walker, 1985) and it is interesting to note the wide use of Progoff's Intensive Journal in religious communities. Elements of the work with the Intensive Journal particularly lend themselves to spiritual exploration both in the depth of working and the structures of the exercises. The way in which Progoff describes the Intensive Journal could be said to generate a sense of depth, an air of mystique or reverence – that is well borne out in the atmosphere of an Intensive Journal workshop.

In a somewhat similar manner to Progoff, Wolf Moondance (1994) describes the use of spirit journals to provide a record of feelings and a place for the recording of dreams in the learning of native American spirit medicine. She describes ways of deepening the sense of ownership of the journal with pictures, beads, sequins. She suggests that the material of dreams, memories, and other recording should be done in paragraphs, not half-sentences, because 'you'll need to make sense of what is being said to you' by 'the inner self... in the spirit world' (1994: 21). The entries should be dated, with the time noted, and a brief reference to the place in which the writing is done ('a little bit about what is going on around you' (1994: 21)). She talks of the need to revere the journal, taking care of it and carrying it – 'Your respect for the journal is very important. It teaches you respect for yourself' (1994: 21). Interestingly, the sense of powerful ownership, of deep personal valuing of the writing process in a journal that these words portray, is no stranger to me as a western European keeper of a personal journal. It does feel bound up intimately with myself.

Part III

Practical issues in journal writing

Chapter 7

Starting to write a learning journal

Introduction

For some, writing reflectively in a journal is no problem. They take to it like the proverbial duck and her water. Some, however, struggle (Dart *et al*, 1998). They want more structure or writing in this way feels unfamiliar; it may feel 'wrong' because their training since school has been to write more formally, not, for example, using the first person. The demise of letter writing may have something to do with the difficulty because a letter to a friend can be similar to a journal entry in style and experience of writing.

This chapter has an important place in this book, not only because of the difficulties of the learners, but because of the difficulty that some teaching staff have with the use of learning journals with their students. It is not unlikely that their difficulties are for the same reasons as those of the writers.

Beyond this introductory section, this chapter considers how to start to write a learning journal from several angles. We look at issues in the management of journal writing, at ways of presenting the task of journal writing and of getting learners started; at ways of improving writing and at some of the difficulties that may be encountered. The sections draw from a review of the literature and from the map of reflective writing (Figure 2.1) and provide a basis for those who might plan to use or to introduce journal writing, or for those who might want to start a journal for themselves.

The management of journal writing

This section largely refers to the management of journal writing in formal educational situations, but some elements will apply to the learner's self-management.

In the preparation of this book, a number of situations have become evident where journals have been introduced without much **forethought**. This can work. It is almost in the nature of journal writing to be experimental – but some thought may mean that the exercise is more likely to be sustained, with a more substantial and satisfying outcome. However, while forethought is important, it is unlikely that a journal will be 'right' the first year. Journal writing evolves with the experiences of the learners and the teaching staff (Ashbury, Fletcher and Birtwhistle, 1993). A first consideration in the management of a task is **the purpose** of the task. Chapter 3 reviewed many purposes for which journals have been used, or that they have fulfilled. Being clear as to why a journal task is set lays the basis for planning, for inducting learners into the task, for the structure (if any) of the journal and for assessment. The aim needs to be made clear to anyone concerned in the project. The aim and the intended journal task also need **to fit within course design**. Creme (1998) indicates that the level of integration of a journal task within a programme is likely to be an influence on its success.

One manner of hinting at the purpose of a journal is represented in **the title** that it is given. We discussed some of the terms used to describe learning journals in Chapter 1, and some relevant generalizations were made about the forms of journals in Chapter 3. The title may generally indicate the type of activity involved in keeping the journal such as in Creme's three examples (Chapter 4) of a 'project journal', a 'record of study' and the 'death journal'.

The management of journal writing involves anticipation of the tasks involved and the demands that may arise from it. **Managing demands** from a small class is very different from managing the demands from a large class and there are some recommendations in the literature that the journals are best suited to small groups of learners who are relatively mature (Stephani, 1997; Hettich, 1990). On the other hand, there are plenty of examples of the relatively sophisticated use of journals in classes of young children (eg Mayher, Lester and Pradl, 1983). A significant variable in management of journals is the degree of monitoring and assessment that are planned. Reading journals may be more enjoyable than reading essays (November, 1993) but it can take a long time, particularly if feedback is (rightly) required. One method of time-saving feedback is that on audiotape.

A reason why journal writing may, in some ways, be easier with young children is because **trust** and **assessment** may be less sensitive issues. Journal writing will work best in an atmosphere of trust (Mayher *et al*, 1983). If the environment is not supportive, it is likely to be the environment that becomes the topic of journal writing. Older students, who are aware of the potential consequences of assessment, need assurance that there is relaxation of concern for the usual elements of writing that matter, such as spelling, construction, and use of formal language. But there will be concerns about the manner in which journals will be monitored or assessed, particularly among students who are not even sure on what they are expected to write however many times this may have been explained (Francis, 1995).

Trust is an issue also for staff. By setting up an openness in the learning situation, Wetherell and Mullins (1996) suggest that 'they expose themselves to criticism in students' journals. They cannot be defensive, or take offence. They must deal with

student criticism, which may be misdirected or unfounded, without aggravating the situation, and in a way that leads to a positive resolution'. Trust between staff and students is important also because journal writing can generate unexpected emotions. Such writing can 'pose a threat to the writer by revealing what lies beneath carefully constructed defenses' (Mayher *et al*, 1983: 34). Similarly, writing can initiate dramatic changes in learner life patterns (Moon, 1999a). There are, for example, stories of students who leave courses after they have the opportunity to explore their feelings in a journal (eg Cooper, 1991). This event may be positive for the individual, but it involves considerable management skills on the part of staff.

Clearly the issue of assessment relates to the trust atmosphere. If learners are required to write journals that are not judged by another, the trust issue is different from situations in which journals are overseen by staff, and different again from those in which journals are graded. Where journals are read, the issue of **privacy or confidentiality** emerges and to some extent, the more that the learners trust the staff member, the more they are likely to feel comfortable about revealing. Methods of managing the privacy of journals are described in the next section.

Where journals are used for **assessment** and where the marks are significant, not only is the openness of the writers potentially under greater threat but they may write according to what they think the assessor wants. We have described the example of students who decided that 'self-flagellation' was what their tutors wanted to read about (Salisbury, 1994). Assessing, but also allowing learners to feel sufficient freedom for expression in a manner that benefits their learning and the purposes of the journal, requires subtle management. Unfortunately, however, a decision not to assess may mean that the journal is not written.

One issue about assessment that does not arise in Chapter 8 is the **possible influence on journal writing of different staff**. We suggested above that students may have different attitudes to journal writing – some may be more and some less able to write reflectively and their ability may not correlate with their aptitude in their studies. Staff, however, may vary in their sympathy for and comprehension of the task of journal writing (Salisbury, 1994). It is not unlikely that students writing a journal for the same purpose may receive very different qualities of feedback from different members of staff overseeing or even marking equivalent work. Mayher *et al* (1983) advise teachers who are overseeing journals: '... be relaxed. Don't overwhelm students with the task, but allow it to develop organically, letting it work for them in ways they discover. By encouraging and gently prodding ... journal writing can open up new learning channels in your curriculum'(1983: 25).

Time is an issue in journal writing for staff and learners. We have said earlier that it is an advantage of journal writing that it creates an intellectual space for learners, but equally, it is the time that it takes that is a major reason for the abandonment of journal writing. The time issue needs to be managed. Some apparently successful journals arise from regular opportunities to write either at the beginning or at the end of classes, sometimes responding to the class content (eg Hahnemann, 1986). However, it is possible that the classroom is not the place that is most conducive to reflection and some teaching staff would argue that they need all of the time available for teaching (and not, they seem to suggest, for helping students to learn!).

Time, of course, relates to the cost–benefit sum. While there are some reports of the **evaluation** of journal writing in the literature, it is probable that the analysis of the benefits for students against the 'cost' in terms of time, staff and student effort is mostly a 'gut feeling'. A problem with any evaluation process is how to choose the criteria against which to evaluate the exercise, and this takes us back to purpose as well as on to assessment.

Presenting the task

Another major aspect of management is how to guide the students, what to tell them, how to get them started. This is the subject of the next section.

Medium for journals

Journals do not need to be on paper. An early decision to be made is the medium for recording. There are advantages and disadvantages in all. Electronic methods, such as e-mail, are very easy to communicate to another who has compatible equipment. There may be no apparent reason why a journal should not be word-processed – though there is evidence that writing on a computer has different qualities from those of writing in hand (Bunker and Cronin, 1997). These may not be the wrong qualities. Recording on audiotape is quick, but it is less easy to 'flick though' or review and there are suggestions that it tends to consist more of descriptive than reflective work (Ficher, 1990). Video could also have possibilities; however, generally speaking and in the rest of this book, we refer to paper-based writing.

Format

Unless there are reasons for prescribing a particular format, it is desirable that the format of a journal is a matter of personal experiment and choice for the learner because this is a manner though which a sense of ownership – a relationship to the writing – is developed. Rainer (1978) points out how the 'rigid design of those one- and five-year' calendar styles of diary influence the manner of writing. There is a specific space to fill and pages of emptiness ahead (James and Denley, 1993). There is advantage in an unstructured format, and, from the point of view of flexibility, even more advantage in using loose-leaf arrangements. Loose-leaves can be written independently from the journal itself and added, enhancing portability. Leaves, however, can also be torn out! Size of the journal may be an issue. Rainer suggests that small books may produce a 'compressed writing style', while they have obvious advantages for portability (Grumet, 1990). Holly mentions the durability of journals. A flimsily covered journal has no chance of lasting for long. With a hard cover, the journal will last and the cover frees the writer from the need to seek other surfaces for support when writing. The format of a journal may be required to provide space for feedback or contributions from another. Wagenaar (1984) asks his students to leave one sheet of each double entry blank for the comments of tutors. Chapter 9 includes some personal observations on journal format.

General instructions

There are instructions that are either helpful or essential when a journal task is first given. Most of them require some decision making in advance and many can be given on a sheet of 'guidelines'. Several writers provide useful lists of instructions (eg Walker, 1985; Fulwiler, 1986; Salisbury, 1994), but most of the content of the lists will be covered in this section or the next which focuses on the improvement of journal technique. The points below are roughly sequenced from those that will require to be followed, to points that provide helpful guidance.

The **purpose of the journal** and the explanation of why the journal task is being set: journals are often 'just given' in a programme. After a year or two of use, they become part of the 'wallpaper' – just like lectures, seminars and essays. More than the other structures of a programme, it is important to tell students why they are being asked to write, what they might expect to get out of the experience and how the purpose relates to the format, design, guidelines and, in particular, any assessment tasks.

For more mature learners, it may be useful to provide some **theory** about the way in which journal writing might enhance their learning or professional development. Journal writing is often used, for example, to enhance reflectiveness in practice. It is helpful for the journal to be introduced alongside this theory and it may be appropriate to talk about the way in which journal writing can support deep learning. Another area of theory with which it is appropriate to introduce journal writing is that of the social construction of knowledge (Cell, 1984; Ross, 1989; Grumet, 1990). Learners can then see their work in journals as a form of building personal theory.

There are a number of reports in the literature that indicate that students may find the step from formal academic writing to the personalized writing that is characteristic of journals to be problematic. They may need to be told several times, and possibly guided by feedback as to the **kind of writing that is desirable in a journal** – or more often, what journal writing is generally not appropriate. November (1993) talks of how he needs to wean his students from 'finished productitis' – the need to tidy and conclude writing as is required in an essay. They need to learn that spelling, style, grammar and completion are not necessarily a part of the process of good journal writing.

Whether the journal is **voluntary or compulsory**: learners may be more willing to work on a journal that is 'strongly advised' or 'will enhance your learning', rather than one that is mandatory.

Assessment: the decision to assess or not assess journals is discussed in Chapter 8. If journals are to be assessed, it is fair to learners to tell them in advance how they are to be assessed and to consider the assessment criteria on which the process will be based (Chapter 8). Assessing journals can be time-consuming. One possibility is to mark a certain number of pages or sections only, and to ask learners to decide which those parts should be. They could mark them with yellow sticky notes. They may also need to number pages to facilitate this.

Separate from assessment, there may be other arrangements for **monitoring and providing feedback** on journals. The frequency for reviewing the progress of learners will depend on many variables, including the nature of the feedback that is to be given. Sometimes the learner may be expected to respond to the tutor's comment and a form of dialogue is developed. As a generalization, most journals used with tertiary students seem to be viewed once or twice a semester, though sometimes more frequently. Wagenaar (1984) comments that viewing three times a term is necessary for appropriate provision of feedback. It may, however, be helpful to students to take in their journals more frequently in the early days in order to give them guidance and feedback. The comments made by a tutor may be a useful subject matter for the next entries (Gibbs, 1988).

The issue of **confidentiality** is important in the management of journal writing, but also as guidance for learners. The need for considerations about confidentiality will depend on the purpose of the journal and the sort of material that a learner is likely to write. However, it could be argued that for a journal to impinge significantly on a learner's processes, the exploration of personal and possibly sensitive material is valuable. Monitoring or an assessment process may dissuade a student from engaging at this level. One means of overcoming this problem is to allow learners to tape together pages that they do not wish to be read, but a more effective alternative is to use a loose-leaf format and to suggest that sensitive writing can be removed before assessment processes. Again yellow sticky notes may mark where material is temporarily removed.

Learners may be invited formally or informally to **read or share their journals** with peers. Sharing material can encourage the writers themselves through comments made, but also can also inspire others in the range of their writing. Sharing may be in pre-arranged sessions, but experience suggests that the option to read material to another, as opposed to paraphrasing it, should be a decision for the student. We consider more formal arrangements for peer support in the section on 'Improving journal writing'.

Chapter 3 introduced a range of possible **structures for journals**. Learners may need instruction on how to use the structure (eg double entry) before they start. As was mentioned earlier, structure can be a means of helping learners to start writing as well as a means to ensure that their reflection 'moves on'. It is not unusual for structures to be suggested but not mandatory – or learners may be asked to start with a given structure and then to design a structure of journal that suits them. We review some structures that are particularly helpful for the initiation of journals further on in this section.

Structures may not emanate from the journal, but may arise as a consequence of the manner in which a journal task is set. For example, Hahnemann (1986) describes how her (nursing) students are asked to write in their journals at the beginning of a class for around 10 minutes. There are also pauses during lectures for writing. Brief assignments are given such as 'write for five minutes on what you have learned about group processes'. The students are also given topics for brief reflection at home.

The material content of a journal: we have tended to consider the content of a journal as writing but depending on the purpose for a journal, other material may be appropriate. There is, for example, no clear division between journals and portfolios where much other material may be presented and linked by reflective writing. Learners may be asked to include academic papers or newspaper articles on which they are asked to reflect. Drawings or photographs or other graphic material may take a principal role in some journals – or a supporting role in others. Wagenaar's sociology students added cartoons or comic strips to illustrate points that they wished to make (Wagenaar, 1984).

It is worth remembering that there are different forms of writing and the use of a variety of forms can greatly enhance the benefits of journals. Poetry, lists, concept-maps and other forms interrogate the writer's capacity in different ways that enhance learning. Chapter 10 describes other such forms that have their place in journals.

The length of a journal or the entries in it is not a measure of the quality of the learning that might result from it. Clearly very brief writing, that does no more than fulfil the minimum requirements, probably results in little learning. Few seem to give indications of how much learners should write. There are several comments, however, on the variation in the amount that is written. Burnard (1988) talks about receiving full A4/letter size binders or a few pages for similar journal tasks from the same group.

The frequency of writing entries probably does require guidance. The instruction to write weekly seems to be common (eg Ghaye and Lillyman, 1997; Burnard, 1988), though Morrison (1990) suggests a minimum limit of twice a term. He also advises students not to try to write up their journals 'at the last moment' before they are handed in. The instruction on the frequency of writing may be modified by suggestions that students keep more regular notes in a notebook to facilitate their writing. Alternatively there might be instructions to learners to reread their entries regularly and to make further comments as a result (eg Ghaye and Lillyman, 1997).

The 'when' and 'where' of writing a journal is likely to be dictated by the nature of the task set. It is worth noting, however, that the format of a journal can dictate when and where it is written more than any other factor. The possibility of writing in a handbag- or pocket-sized journal makes the activity more flexible than the use of essentially a non-transportable journal. The ability to write at any time can be liberating.

Sometimes it is worth thinking about the **audience** in writing a journal. Gibbs' students, who wrote comments about journal writing, considered that identification of an audience may 'allow you to give direction to your thinking' (Gibbs, 1988: 99). The writing may not be for the self. Even if the other 'audience' does not, in reality, see the journal, the sense of audience will influence the manner of writing. Elbow and Clarke make this point strongly: 'An audience is a field of force. The closer we come, the more we think about these readers – the stronger the pull they exert over the contents of our minds' (1987: 19). We have raised the unfortunate possibility that the audience is simply the tutor. Otherwise the writing might be for peers, for a grandchild (Rainer, 1978), for a mentor or an imaginary figure. Holly (1991) comments that when she writes material for others, 'I am more able to speak clearly (and concisely) to the topic'. If the 'audience' is, indeed, self, then it is worth thinking about which self – the self now or the self in the future when the journal might be reread.

Ways of getting started – using the map of reflective writing as a teaching tool

We have suggested that some learners will have no difficulty in getting started on writing in a journal, but others will seem, perhaps, not to understand the task. They will not know what to write about or how to write differently from other academic tasks. The map of reflective writing may be helpful here (Figure 2.1). It can be used to indicate to them the processes involved in reflective writing. It will, in effect, produce a structure that they can use while they need it, and can discard when they have become more confident. A handout or session will be required in which the headings and the components or activities that they encompass are introduced. An initial exercise might then be to plot out a process of reflection (or potential journal entry) under the headings. A summary of the headings in Figure 2.1 appears below:

Description

- observation;
- comment on personal behaviour;
- comment on reaction or feelings;
- comment on context etc.

Additional ideas

- further observation;
- relevant other knowledge, experience, feelings, intuitions;
- suggestions from others;
- new information;
- formal theory;
- other factors such as ethical, moral, socio-political context etc.

Reflective thinking occurs

- processes of relating, experimenting, exploring, reinterpreting from different points of view; or within different contextual factors, theorizing, linking theory and practice; 'cognitive housekeeping', etc.

Other processing such as testing of ideas in practice and/or representation such as in a first draft or graphic form/in discussion.

A product results – something is learned or there is a sense of 'moving on' eg identification of an area for further reflection or a new question is framed.

Either there is more reflection –
or there is resolution or completion

Other ways of getting started

There are a number of other ways of introducing journal writing that are described in the literature. Some are completely compatible with the use of the map (above). Elbow makes a suggestion that seems to underpin all of these methods:

> The secret of getting words down on paper is learning to adopt a casual attitude that is new for most people, a sense of trust that when you have the germ of an idea or even just the hankering for one, you will be led, sooner or later, to the words you are looking for if you just start in writing.
>
> (Elbow, 1981: 47)

Some consider that **free writing techniques** are a valuable means of starting. The writers are encouraged simply to write for a certain length of time – whatever comes into their minds, feelings, thoughts, observations, anything (Rainer, 1978). The results are probably best treated as an exercise increasing the flow of writing, though free writing may be developed as part of a longer exercise (Yinger and Clark, 1981).

Questions are widely used as a means of starting journal writers. It is much easier to answer a question than to generate new material. Questions may guide the journal writer's sequence of thinking (Carlsmith, www), and Johns (1994) developed a set of questions for nurse education which focus on reactions to and actions following from an event that has occurred. Morrison (1990, 1996) developed several sets of questions to aid the reflective processes of teacher education students. The questions guide the process of journal writing so that initially there is a focus on describing, then on organizing and reviewing the material and finally on analysis of, and reflection on, the material.

Other techniques of initiating journal writing follow work on theoretical constructs such as **the Kolb cycle of experiential learning or questionnaires on learning styles**. There are also several descriptions of the use of autobiographical tasks as a starting point for journals (eg Knowles, 1993; November, 1993). Bolton and Styles (1995) give a useful account of an autobiography workshop.

It seems particularly helpful to **show students examples of well-constructed journals**, perhaps from previous students (eg Redwine, 1989). Wagenaar (1984) suggests that examples of good journals are put on reserve in a library together with comments from the tutor. An alternative to this is to ask students at the end of the year to **write advice to students** who will be starting journals in the following year, such as descriptions by Walker (1985) and Gibbs (1988). The engineering students described by Gibbs did this by brainstorming on ideas for advice. They shared out the ideas for a writing-up stage and then circulated the notes for comment. The advice was then made available for other students. The advice given in these two papers is addressed to the learners and it includes the following:

- **Make it your own** – The journal is 'an extension of yourself, not something outside of you', its usefulness 'can be in proportion to the extent to which it is your own' (Walker, 1985: 54).
- **Be honest** – 'Be frank and honest in your entries' (Walker, 1985: 55).
  'You can only learn from your journal if you have enough courage to face

yourself as you really are' (Gibbs, 1988: 99).

- **Let words flow** – 'Write about whatever is at the top of your mind' (Gibbs, 1988: 98).

  '... get down to it ... write, write, write ... let it flow, uncensored and in whatever order it comes. It is very useful simply to write and then to reflect on what has been written' (Walker, 1985: 55).

  'Once you have got going, ideas will tend to lead on to other ideas and before you know it, you will be into your journal'(Gibbs, 1988: 98).

- **Use your own words – be informal** – '... use simple English that makes you realize exactly what you meant when you review your journal' (Gibbs, 1988: 98).

  '... use your own words, put your own name on things. Say what you feel, and if that makes you feel guilty, record that and work with it further' (Walker, 1985: 55).

- **Dig deeper** – 'Urge yourself to keep digging deeper and deeper so that you can understand and use your understanding. Try to work towards "truths" you have discovered through your experiences; (towards) advice to yourself about what to do in the near future; (and towards) finding questions that you need to think about next, about issues which you don't yet fully understand but need to understand' (Gibbs, 1988: 100).

- **Be flexible** – 'Do not be rigid in the way you keep (the journal) ... Be prepared to try different methods, so that you can mould this exercise to your personal talents and needs...' (Walker, 1985: 55).

- **Write things up as soon as you can** – 'There is a very definite advantage in being able to record things as quickly as possible, even though one may not immediately write them up fully'(Walker, 1985: 55).

- **Seek help if necessary** – 'Feel free to seek help ... from others: fellow participants, or other people who have used this type of exercise, or the facilitators of the programme' (Walker, 1985: 56).

- **Be selective** – Walker (1985: 56) suggests that most of the participants recognized that in the beginning they wrote a great deal more than was necessary. 'Selectivity was a sign of experience....'

Improving journal writing

Although this chapter is largely about starting to write journals, we add a few methods that have been used to improve the quality of journals themselves, or of the learning that can result from writing in journals. The use of activities that are described in the last chapter would constitute another method of improving journal writing. The methods presented in this section fall into four groups. The first group involves developments in the journal as a physical entity. The second group consists of a variety of mechanisms to deepen learning (see Chapter 2 for references to deep and surface learning). The third group is represented by a number of theoretical frameworks that can be introduced to deepen learning and the fourth involves taking an overview (meta-view) of learning journal work.

Improving the organization of learning journals

There are various reasons why journal writers might want to think of new ways of organizing their journals. They may be required to refer to it within an essay, for example, and we have suggested above that some, but not all of a journal may be marked, with choice of which parts are to be marked left to the learner. Both of these examples might indicate that the pages of a journal may be numbered, and, perhaps, contents listed. It might be appropriate to divide writing into sections – structuring the journal like a double entry journal, for example (Chapter 3). Progoff's Intensive Journal provides ideas for many other sections.

Other methods of organizing journal writing – perhaps one could say 'making the journal work better for you' – involve emphasizing, making headings, highlighting and marking in cross-references. Cross-references might be identified by symbols, icons, colour, stickers, coloured paper and so on. The use of different pens or different colours can enable a different form of self-expression. Holly (1991) comments that sometimes 'red "feels" right; at other times it's green'. She suggests also that comments might be made in the margin in different colours at a later reread. It is possible to underline or circle (Walker, 1985), to use arrows and asterisks and even to cut and paste (Voss, 1988). Allied to these forms of marking might be techniques, suggested by Progoff (1975), of summarizing periods of time or events in a single image.

Deepening learning

Methods of deepening learning from the process of journal writing are likely to involve the use of an incentive to think more about what has been written or what might be written (November, 1993). We have suggested that questions are useful to help learners at the start of journal writing. Different, more prompting questions have value also in deepening the processing in a journal. Morrison's (1996) paper provides some useful examples.

Methods that involve the encouragement of learners to reread and reflect further on what they have written in earlier entries are likely also to enhance deeper learning (Walker, 1985; Ghaye and Lillyman, 1997). Apart from the use of methods like double entry journals, assessment tasks that require learners to draw from their journals demand rereading and the rethinking of entries. Several of these techniques could be combined to deepen learning if learners are asked to reconsider the content of their journals in terms of their implications for social, ethical or other contextual issues (Heath, 1998) that, we have suggested, engage deeper processing.

Brockbank and McGill (1998) develop another group of methods of promoting deeper processing in a comprehensive manner. They believe that the key to useful reflection is facilitation by another. An example of this is the use of 'critical friends' who are described by Francis (1995) as particularly significant in increasing the skills of reflection of teaching students. Her students worked in pairs or small groups, within the agenda set by their partners. They aimed to 'stimulate, clarify and extend thinking within their framework of beliefs, values and needs'. They found it 'difficult but exciting'. Sagor (1991) lists some useful guidelines for 'critical friends', many of which concern the important issues of interests and agendas.

The development of peer and self-assessment for journals (Chapter 8), where the learners have some part in the judgement of appropriate criteria, is another method which tends to promote deeper learning (Burnard, 1988; Mortimer, 1998). Learners are more involved with their work and understand better what they are trying to do. Self-assessment is illustrated in Hettich's work (described below).

The introduction of theoretical frameworks to deepen processing

Several writers report the introduction to students of existing frameworks that describe aspects of cognitive function. Hettich (1990) refers to 'attempting to "stretch" the (journal writing) technique' with his psychology students. Halfway through the courses he introduced the cognitive domain of Bloom's (1956) taxonomy of educational objectives. He suggested that the students should analyse their previous entries for the level of function indicated. The basic level is knowledge, then comprehension, application, analysis, synthesis and evaluation. He asked them to indicate the level of subsequent entries and generally to avoid 'knowledge'. Evaluating the results of a pilot investigation of this, Hettich says, 'Typically, students wrote at higher and more diverse levels of Bloom's hierarchy once they understood and correctly applied the taxonomy.' Joyce (www) also describes the application of Bloom's work to journals – initially for assessment and then to develop their critical thinking.

Hettich went on to consider whether the introduction of other frameworks of cognitive function might encourage students to increase the sophistication of their work in journals. He introduced the model of Perry (1970) to students though a lecture and handout and asked them to analyse their journal entries in the same way. They were interested in the model but 'found it difficult to understand when applied to journal entries' (Hettich, 1990). Hettich suggests that the model of Belenky *et al* (1986) may have more promise and similarly we suggest that of King and Kitchener (1994). Both are mentioned in Chapter 2. More time and careful planning and monitoring would be needed for their introduction.

Taking a meta-view of learning journal work

The work of Hettich, described above, also provides an example of the fourth group of methods of improving writing in learning from journals. It involves a metacognitive approach. Chapter 2 indicates reasonable evidence that a means by which journals improve learning is through their enhancement of metacognition – the taking of an overview of one's learning processes. This can be exploited in journals by:

- focusing the attention of learners on to their processes of learning as part of the work that they do in the journal;

- like Hettich (1990) – above – by asking them to analyse aspects of their entries for qualities of learning (eg by use of Bloom's taxonomy);
- asking them to review the whole process of keeping a journal in relation to the learning that results from it. There are a number of reports of evaluation of journals (eg Hahnemann, 1986; Wetherell and Mullins, 1996; Ghaye and Lillyman, 1997), but none seem to be focused directly on the intention to improve learning from subsequent journal or reflective writing.

A variation on these methods of meta-viewing of journals, which fits also in the second section on facilitation, is the situation in which staff choose to write journals alongside their students (eg Knowles, 1993; Miller, 1983) and to share entries, particularly those on the processes of journal writing.

Difficulties that may be encountered in journal writing

We have said several times before in several contexts that some learners have difficulty in writing reflectively or in a journal. However, it is possible that those who have the most difficulty in the beginning stand to be those who can gain the most from the exercise (Handley, 1998).

The literature provides a range of reasons why learners might find journal writing difficult. For example: some learners resist, not seeing the relevance of journal writing to their current pursuit (Francis, 1995; Hatton and Smith, 1995); some are cynical or feel that 'reflection' is over-emphasized (James and Denley, 1993; Salisbury, 1994) or concerned that they will not produce what the teacher wants, or they are too concerned to produce what they perceive to be wanted (Dillon, 1983). Many are reported to request more guidance or structure (Ashbury, Fletcher and Birtwhistle, 1993; Heath, 1998; Dart *et al*, 1998). Students on courses often feel that they do not have time to engage in an activity whose value may not be as obvious at the time (Hettich, 1976; Francis, 1995; Anbar, www). They are likely, perhaps misguidedly, to assume that they learn more from traditional approaches to teaching – because they are traditional.

Procrastination on the part of learners is often a problem for the reasons cited in the paragraph above, or for others. Many students have study habits that do not accord with regular journal entries in that they let tasks accumulate and only under pressure make the due effort (Canning, 1991).

Some learners have difficulty in focusing their writing, particularly in the early stages of using a journal. 'Rambling' entries can be a problem, particularly where no structure is provided (Francis, 1995). Some learners recognize the role that rambling around ideas works for them. We have already cited Canning (1991) who reports one of her students as saying 'I just ramble until all of a sudden two or three words will fit together and key something. Then I realize that's it! That's where I'm having the problem! And then I can go with that.' Francis (1995) found those who rambled 'tended to assume stronger ownership of both the journal and the knowledge generated there'.

However, rambling can imply 'going in circles' or taking a superficial approach (Hoover, 1994; Ghaye and Lillyman, 1997). 'Going in circles' is likely to indicate that the learners are not moving through what we have represented as the map of reflective writing (Figure 2.1). They are probably 'stuck' at the stage of descriptive writing and not actually progressing towards reflective thinking processes to reach useful outcomes of learning or more material for reflection. They may need help to understand how to 'move on' through the process – perhaps using the map for guidance.

Journal writing activities may have a good chance of evolving positively but the project may also grow stale and the writing and the management of it may become a chore. This may be the time to put journals aside (Dillon, 1983; Wetherell and Mullins, 1996; Ghaye and Lillyman, 1997) or redesign the whole approach, perhaps using some of the suggestions in the 'Improvements' section earlier in this chapter, or activities from the last chapter.

Chapter 8

Assessing journals and other reflective writing

Introduction

This chapter is primarily concerned about journals used in formal educational situations where it may be usual to assess the work of learners. A key issue that underlies the very writing of this chapter is whether or not journals should be assessed, but first it is necessary to clarify the meaning of 'assessment' as it is to be used here.

Assessment is a word that is used differently in different situations. Assessment is taken to mean here the review of a journal by tutors or perhaps self or peers. The purpose of the review is to indicate how well the journal is matching some criteria for assessment and the information on relative success may be for the learner or for those who are conducting the programme when it can be used for grading or marking purposes. The results of this process may be used to determine the value of the journal as a method of learning and facilitation of learning. In the same way, the measure may be of the degree to which the journal as a method relates to expected learning outcomes or fits with the aims of the programme of learning, but in the context of this chapter, the focus is the learner.

Assessment of journals may be formative or summative. Formative assessment is a means of presenting learners with feedback on their work as they progress with it, whereas summative assessment occurs at the end of the work and provides an overview of the quality of the work, sometimes as a grade or mark.

Should journals be assessed?

There are many that argue that journals and reflective writing should not be assessed. A convinced proponent of journals in drama, Sister Therese Craig, asks:

> How can you mark an individual's own personal development? I think it's a right and proper part of education for us to encourage students to express their feelings so that they know it's all right to have those feelings. However, for me to mark those feelings seems inconsistent and incongruent. Marks can also create a barrier or obstacle to the person finding his or her own voice.
>
> (Dillon, 1983)

Sumsion and Fleet (1996) also question the assessment of reflection in more general terms. They note that there is no evidence that a reflective professional is more effective than a non-reflective professional or that programmes that promote reflection lead to better outcomes. In a series of experiments they sought to explore the issue in their work with final-year early childhood education students (n=124). The students did not work specifically with journals, but with written reflective accounts submitted periodically. They found that they faced the same problem that underlies much of the content of this chapter – that of finding a suitable set of criteria by which to code the 'reflectiveness' of the students' work. They reviewed and rejected a number of instruments. The instruments, some of which are considered later in this chapter, were either too complex for the number of scripts with which they were working, or were composed of too many categories to obtain sufficient inter-coder reliability. They finally used criteria based on Boud, Keogh and Walker (1985). Despite the relative simplicity of their three-point scale – non-reflective, moderately reflective and highly reflective, their inter-coder reliability was only 50 per cent. This low reliability influenced their further conclusion on the relationship between reflective tendencies and academic ability. They concluded that it is possible to be reflective without being academically able.

Sumsion and Fleet's work is useful for the difficult issues that it demonstrates in the assessment of reflection. They say: 'at present, there are substantial difficulties involved in attempting to identify and assess reflection. Given current methodological and pragmatic limitations, the assessment of reflection raises complex issues of consistency and equity, as well as broader pedagogical and ethical concerns.' On the basis of this, they abandoned their attempts to assess reflection.

It is very easy to go along with arguments that assessment of reflective writing or journals is intrusive on personal development or is too difficult – the first, perhaps, more than the second. However, there are reasons why we do need to develop means of assessment while, at the same time, taking a broader view of the process than is taken by either of the papers above. The first reason reiterates the comments made by Sumsion and Fleet. Students are being assessed on journals and reflective writing. Even where journal writing is assessed on the basis of 'competent' or 'not yet competent', or pass or fail/not yet pass, the criteria being used are often 'gut reactions' or personal interpretations. When reflection and reflective practice are so highly esteemed in some areas of education and professional development, we should be able to do better than this. The coders involved in the work of Sumsion and Fleet demonstrated a substantial mismatch in their coding even when working with a simple scheme.

The second justification for a system of assessment is based on the observation that even able learners may not find reflective writing in a journal easy (Wildman and Niles, 1987). Unless teachers have an understanding of the task that they are setting and the qualities in it that constitute a good performance, they will not be able to help these learners. As teachers, their ability to help may be hampered by the likelihood that they are naturally reflective and perhaps less able to recognize the problems of others. The understanding of the task which teachers need in order to be helpful is displayed in the assessment criteria.

A third justification for the assessment of reflective writing is rooted in the nature of the higher education system, as it seems to exist. The rise of the 'strategic' student is well documented (eg Kneale, 1997). 'Strategic students' are intent on success in their studies for the minimum output and will therefore not put effort into tasks that are not assessed. If we believe that journals contribute to learning, then the assessment of journals may be necessary in order to ensure the requisite student effort.

Fourthly, many professional development programmes are based on the development of the reflective practitioner. The nature of the learning outcomes for such programmes should relate to assessment criteria for reflective practice. Reflective practice is very often evidenced in journals or other reflective writing. This reasoning led Hatton and Smith (1995) to research what might constitute 'evidence of reflection'. They concluded that the best evidence for reflection is in written accounts. On this basis they researched and developed a typology of qualities of reflective activity in writing that is described later in this chapter.

The fifth reason for developing methods of assessing journals is the opposite of the tentative justifications above. Students are assessed on their programmes of learning and there is nothing wrong with setting journal writing or similar work as a method of assessment (Paulson, Paulson and Meyer, 1991), and even as a method of grading students. What matters, as elsewhere, is that both we and the students are clear about the criteria for the assessment.

The last point is more general. Assessment does not always mean marking. In the sense that Brockbank and McGill use the term, it can mean 'sitting beside', a collaborative rather than an inspectorial system (Brockbank and McGill, 1998: 100–01). It is a helpful process to learners and it can bring structure and discipline to the work that might not come about in completely unassessed work (Macrorie, 1970).

The points above strongly justify the development of assessment criteria for reflective and journal writing even if they do not argue for the necessity to mark or grade journals under all circumstances. The next section of this chapter follows on from this to consider issues and decisions that contribute to the design of assessment procedures. But an important point is that learning journals are not set for only one purpose. If there are different purposes for writing journals, there will be different ways of assessing them, which will bear a relationship to the purpose for which they are used.

Issues and decisions in the assessment of journals and reflective writing

What is to be assessed – process or product?

This is, perhaps, a big question that is often not asked. Generally speaking, journal writing employs reflective writing in order to support some form of learning. In many situations the learning is what is important, and the reflective writing is a means to that end. For example, Selfe, Petersen and Nahrgang (1986) describe the use of journals with mathematics students. The aim of the work is not to develop reflective skills in these students, but to improve their learning. The quality of their reflection is incidental.

At other times, the quality of the reflective process evidenced in the writing is as or more important than the learning that results. There are many examples in the literature of learning journals used in teacher education where the objective will be to enhance the skills of reflection on practice as well as to bring about learning. The work of Calderhead and James (1992) with the Record of Student Experience (ROSE) exemplifies this approach. While many, perhaps most uses of journal writing will be expected to provide process and product outcomes, clarity about what is expected will guide the development of assessment criteria. In situations where it is the learning that is important, there is much less of a problem with the development of criteria and the procedures. The learning may be evidenced directly in the journal and it is likely to be couched in disciplinary terms (Brockbank and McGill, 1998), or the learning may be assessed indirectly in examinations or other forms of assessment. The complexities of the assessment of journals become evident when there is concern for the process as well as or more than the learning product.

Purpose and the development of assessment criteria

Assessment criteria can be the criteria that will indicate that the journal has reached an adequate standard for acceptance, or they can be graded qualitatively so that they guide the assessor in allocating a grade or mark. In higher education, there may be a set of level descriptors that will guide the level of difficulty with which learners at any particular level will be able to cope. Some of the statements refer to reflective capacity (eg Moon, 1996a). We have suggested that there are many different purposes for asking learners to write journals or to write reflectively. The purpose should be reflected in the assessment criteria and both purpose and assessment criteria will be decided and indicated to students long before the journals are started. For example, if the journal is kept in order to enhance the learning, or metacognitive skills of the learner, the relation of the journal writing to these skills should be explicit. In many situations, teaching staff may not be clear as to the purpose for which they set journal writing. Sometimes the journal method seems like 'a good idea'. It does not, therefore, make entire sense to suggest that the purpose must be influential in consideration of the assessment criteria.

The reality of the situation in which journals come to be assessed is that assessment time is looming, and journals need to be marked but there is overt or covert indecision as to how to mark them. In the end they are marked according to 'gut feelings'. Gut feelings are personal criteria that the learners will never know, and which may not match across all of those who mark. Much of this chapter is about the development of assessment criteria that can be made explicit and agreed to be a fair means of judging journal or reflective writing.

Purposes and assessment criteria do not always have to be developed by the tutor. Some or all of the criteria may be developed by the learners on the basis of their perception of the purpose and the nature of the task. This might be in addition to criteria already made explicit by the tutor. Alternatively peer groups might determine criteria. A number of examples later in this chapter demonstrate reliance on assessment criteria implied by particular models or views of reflection. For clarity it is important that the development of assessment criteria is seen as a separate operation to the process of making a judgement of the journal against the criteria. It would, for example, be possible for a tutor to judge journals against criteria set by a peer group of learners – or by the writers themselves. Various combinations are demonstrated in the examples later in the chapter. Involvement of learners in decisions about assessment criteria creates a sense of ownership of work, and a greater awareness of the nature of the task, its purpose and its potential for their learning.

Direct and indirect assessment

Assessment of journals does not automatically imply that the journals themselves are reviewed. There are several examples given below where assessment is indirect in that a task that is based on the journal is assessed instead of the journal itself.

The effects of assessing journals

The decision to assess journals has a number of implications. If the assessment is direct and the teacher sees the journal material itself, there is immediately a problem for the learners if they want to write about personal issues. Ways of managing privacy in journals have been described in Chapter 7 and we have also noted the manner in which assessment of journals may influence the content of a journal. This is possibly to the detriment of the journal.

The management of assessment of journals

Assessment without direct grading

Assessment of journals does not automatically imply that the journal is allocated a grade. There are a number of alternatives to consider even in a modular system and bearing in mind the need to motivate the strategic student (see above). Firstly, the submission of a journal that meets some general characteristics of completeness and quality of presentation may be deemed essential for progression to the next modules, semester or year of study. Similar to this in its effect is the allocation of a single and fairly high mark to all journals that are adequate, with inadequate journals being returned for further work. A slightly more elaborate method is to use a system of three grades with simple assessment criteria such as length and regularity of entry distinguishing between them (eg Brodsky and Meagher, 1987). A different but equally simple approach is used by Jensen (1987) for physics students. The students were told that a well-kept journal, with quantity as the main criterion, could improve their semester course grade by up to a third of a grade point (eg from C to C+). This served to motivate 90 per cent of the students.

The assessment of journals within the context of a programme

Where marks are allocated to journals, there is a decision as to what percentage of the total programme or module mark will be given to the journal. There are a number of comments about this in the literature. Often those who have allocated a low percentage (for example around 10 per cent) have done so initially in order to ensure that journals are kept (Hahnemann, 1986). However, it appears to be relatively common for these percentages to be increased, sometimes quite dramatically, as the assessors have become more confident of the journal's contribution to learning and of their own ability to assess such work. For example, Brodsky and Meagher shifted percentages of course marks in a political science programme from 10 per cent to 25 per cent to 75 per cent, having moved from initially seeing journals as an 'adjunct to, rather than an integral part of the courses' (1987: 375). In a similar state of uncertainty about the method for his commerce students, November (1993) initially assigned 15 per cent of marks to journals. A year later he assigned 40 per cent of the final mark to journals, reducing essay and project work, and a year later again he abandoned all other assessment, making the journal account for the total mark for his course. Taking a different approach, Hettich (1990) asked his students what percentage of total psychology course grades should be allocated to journal writing. The median report was 25 per cent, which suggested that they preferred to see the journal as a 'supplement to other measures of learning'.

Coping with the volume of reading in the assessment of journals

An important issue in assessing journals is the matter of coping with the volume of reading. If the assessment is formative as well as summative, journals will be handed in for perusal and comment on a regular basis. It may be necessary to advise students either to restrain the volume of their writing, or to summarize material where original entries have been extensive. One mechanism that neatly overcomes the problem of reading volume is to ask learners to identify particular areas for assessment within the context of a complete journal. This means that they have the opportunity to identify what they consider to be their best work, and the assessor reads less while being aware of the full journal. Houghton (1998) uses an approach of this type in a module on learning from work experience.

Formative assessment – the provision of feedback

The provision of feedback or the making of comments on journals requires greater sensitivity than other situations of marking. Sister Craig's comment about her students' feelings in the second section of this chapter epitomizes the issue. Cowan (1998b) suggests some very helpful guidelines for making sensitive comments on student journal entries:

- avoid writing comments in the first person in order to avoid setting up dialogue between writers and tutor when the dialogue should be between writers and themselves;
- avoid suggestion of judgements – provide an opportunity for writers to judge for themselves if it seems appropriate;
- ask a question or make a comment about a non-sequitur when it is useful to seek clarification;
- make a note when one wants to react negatively or positively to journal material but make no comment; however,
- indicate where more thinking could be appropriate or helpful.

Cowan stresses the responsibility of the assessor in overlooking journal material. The material should be treated as confidential and not discussed elsewhere.

In addition to the possibly sensitive quality of the material in a journal, the purposes for which most journals are written would suggest a sense of ownership within which teacher comments may be physical impositions. Writing comments in pencil can partially overcome this. Another method is to use yellow sticky notes or a page of comments referenced into the journal. Essential for this to work would be clearly numbered pages or sections. Commenting on an audio-cassette tape is another useful possibility. This is a technique that is under-exploited for commenting on any assessed work.

Self and peer assessment

As in other forms of assessment, journals do not have to be assessed by a tutor. Sometimes it will be appropriate for the learner or a group of learners either to decide the criteria that should be the basis for assessment or to mark against given criteria, or to conduct both operations. Such situations may be more likely in the context of self-directed work or where personal development is the purpose, or in more general situations with mature learners.

Development of assessment criteria may also be a joint process between staff and learners. Burnard (1988) suggests a method by which this may be done. Tutor and student 'brainstorm' criteria for assessment and from the list, each use the criteria in order to assess the journal and they make notes in support of their decisions. A discussion follows and a mark can be produced as a result of the discussion if necessary. This method could be the basis of many variations. One variation, which makes better use of the process in terms of learning, would be to undertake the development of criteria when the learners have spent a short while (out of the projected time) writing the journal. In this way, they will have some experience of the process before criteria are decided, and then can use the criteria as a guide to the rest of their work on the journal.

Assessment of journals and reflective writing – some examples

The examples described below represent approaches to assessment and some different sets of assessment criteria that have been used for the process. In many cases, when an approach is described in the literature, there are no details given of the assessment criteria. In the design of assessment for journals, it is important that both approach and criteria should be considered, though sometimes the approach is no more than the marking of journals against assessment criteria. The major divisions in this review of assessment mechanisms for journals are:

- indirect approaches to assessment;
- approaches to the development of assessment criteria;
- assessment criteria developed from the work of others;
- 'purpose-made' assessment tools.

Indirect approaches to the assessment of journals

Indirect approaches are described in an earlier section as the assessment of work on the subject matter of the journal, not on the journal itself. Some advantages of the indirect approaches are that they can force learners to review and reconsider the contents of their journals, and to link them to theory, and they may thereby encourage greater learning from the journal. They are also more controllable in terms of the volume of reading or time taken for assessment. As well as the use of an indirect approach to summative assessment of journals, tutors may choose to provide formative assessment by discussing the content of journals with learners.

The interview or viva. The learners are interviewed about the contents of their journal. The examiners may have read the journal or may relate their questions to the material on which the journal is based. Martin (1998) has suggested that in this kind of interview, the more the learners are able to take control of the conversation, the more ability they are demonstrating in reflection.

Lindberg (1987) describes what he calls a 'conference' with his English literature students. The three conferences on the course are one to one, and they last around 15 or 20 minutes. Lindberg describes them to his students:

> Since the journal is your gesture of making meaning, I will not grade it directly or read through it systematically. Instead, I want to respond to your own responses to what is going on in the journal. You'll summarize for me the high points of your journal and interpret yourself as an interpreter. And I'll probably ask you some hard questions about your responses and name for you what I see in your summary.
>
> Lindberg (1987: 121)

He goes on to describe a longer (half-hour) conference at the end of the course in which performance is graded. The grade counts for a third of the marks of the course and the rest is made up of interpretive essays, which often relate to the material of the journal.

An essay based on the content of the journal. Students are told at the start of their journal work that they will be required to write an essay based on their journals. They may or may not be given the title and they may or may not be given the assessment criteria for the essay. Morrison (1996) uses this approach in postgraduate teacher education. An example of an assignment is 'With reference to appropriate literature, experiences through the course, your personal professional context and to the Learning Log, evaluate the notion of progression in learning' (Morrison, 1990).

Students are required to make reference to the material in their journals in other coursework. This may be explicitly introduced through learning outcomes that refer to journal work.

A rewritten version of the journal. The rewritten accounts may be structured by guidelines – for example, to summarize the areas of significant reflection, and present the thoughts or new learning that emerge more formally.

Questions for further consideration. Learners are required to identify questions that are raised by their journal work that require further reflection or investigation. The quality of the questions is as important as their subject matter. The work of Morgan and Saxon (1991) on the structure of questions would support this exercise.

Approaches to the development of assessment criteria

Among references to assessment criteria that are of relevance to the assessment of journals or reflective writing, there appear to be several groupings. The first grouping consists of informal ideas, often in the form of guidance given to students. Secondly, there are more formal attempts to develop classifications for grading of quality and lastly there are several uses of models developed for different purposes, but now applied to assessment of reflective accounts (eg Bloom's taxonomy and the SOLO taxonomy). Some of the criteria below are indications of adequacy or competent performance and some are graded to enable a mark to be allocated.

Some general criteria that can helpfully indicate adequacy. These criteria are derived from a range of sources in the literature, in particular Hettich (1976), Wagenaar (1984), Fulwiler (1987), November (1993) and Newman (www). Most journals will need to demonstrate quality in at least some of the following:

- length;
- presentation and legibility;
- number of entries or regularity of entries;
- clarity and good observation in presentation of events or issues;
- evidence of speculation;
- evidence of a willingness to revise ideas;
- honesty and self assessment*;
- thoroughness of reflection and self-awareness;
- depth and detail of reflective accounts;
- evidence of creative thinking;
- evidence of critical thinking;
- a deep approach to the subject matter of the journal;
- representation of different cognitive skills (synthesis, analysis, evaluation etc);
- relationship of the entries in the journal to any relevant coursework, theories, etc;
- match of the content and outcomes of the journal work to course objectives, learning outcomes for the journal or purposes that the journal is intended to fulfil;
- questions that arise from the reflective processes and on which to reflect further.

*('Final reports always read as if everything had gone according ... to plan. ... You come up against problems, struggle with them and finally overcome them. Learning journals should reveal this process' (Newman, www).)

Assessment criteria developed from the work of others

While some of the schema below might seem attractive means to assess journal work, it is worth recalling the difficulties encountered by Sumsion and Fleet when they tried to use some more complex criteria for assessment of reflective accounts.

Criteria based on Bloom's taxonomy of educational objectives. Hettich (1976, 1990), using journals in the context of psychology courses, uses Bloom's (1956) taxonomy both as subject matter for the journal and as a means of analysis of the entries. This is described in Chapter 7. Hettich speculated that other models of thinking such as those of Perry (1970) and Belenky *et al* (1986) might also contribute to the understanding of journal work. In the publication on reflection (Moon, 1999a), I review these models of thinking in relation to the concept of reflection. The review includes also the model of King and Kitchener (1994) – to which reference is made below (and in Chapter 2).

Criteria based on King and Kitchener's model of reflective judgement. Ross (1989) developed a set of criteria for a teacher education programme. The criteria were not specifically developed to assess journal writing, but various forms of reflective activities. Ross found that the seven-stage model of Kitchener and King (1981 – updated version, 1994) provides a good basis for development of criteria for assessing levels of reflection. The criteria are very much related to teacher education, but elements are extracted or summarized below in a more generalized manner.

Level 1
- Observes teacher implementing (or not so doing) research finding – little analysis, little reasoning, supporting comment or concern for impact on learners.
- Poor ability to integrate observation of teacher behaviour with research principle, eg focusing on only one aspect of the behaviour or the research.
- In reading an article, restates ideas of the article; cannot adapt the ideas in the article to the more constrained environment of the real classroom. Stresses single solutions to problems.

Level 2
- Can describe situations well, but does not take into account the multiplicity of factors that can underlie an event. Limited in perspectives.
- Can analyse differences in practice and good and poor practice, but cannot conduct the reasoning that explains the differences.
- Is not clear about the influences of various factors on which teaching strategies are based.

Level 3
- 'Views things from multiple perspectives'; can cope with conflicting aims, different personal perspectives, the role of context in educational decisions etc.
- Can comprehend the pervasive impact of teaching beyond the point of instruction.

Ross makes some observations that seem to be relevant to the experiences of others who have set up assessment criteria. She comments on the time taken for marking and suggests that the assessor needs to be familiar with the material on which the students are reflecting in order to know whether their thoughts are original or those of another. The assessor in this case felt that the students would have been able to reflect at a higher level if they had understood more about the nature of reflection and the criteria on which they were to be assessed.

Assessment based on the Structure of Learning Outcomes (SOLO) taxonomy. The SOLO taxonomy (Biggs and Collis, 1982) was developed as a means of describing the outcomes of learning and it has been used in a number of different contexts (eg Moon, 1999a). Davies (1998) used SOLO as a means of assessing student reports of art and design projects.

The model consists of five levels that appear to be relatively easily recognized in written material. In Level 1 work (Prestructural), there is no appropriate structure to the task. The second level is Unistructural, with only one general element taken into account. In the third (Multistructural) level, there are several elements present in the representation but they are presented in an unrelated or poorly integrated manner. In the Relational – fourth – level, the several elements are integrated coherently in such a way that a new structure can be identified, but this new structure is not readily generalized to new situations. At the most sophisticated level – that of the Extended Abstract – the developed new structure is flexibly and competently generalized to new situations. It is interesting to note that there are elements of the SOLO taxonomy that correspond to Ross's work and that of King and Kitchener (see above). Ross describes her level-one reflection as limited to a single dimension with inability to analyse beyond. At her second level, students are able to recognize the existence of different influences on a situation, but are not able to integrate them in planning or anticipation of consequences. At her highest level, Ross describes the reflective capacity in terms of comprehension and ability to work with multiple perspectives and their multiple influences on a situation.

Assessment based on Van Manen's levels of reflectivity. Wedman and Martin (1986) used Van Manen's three schemata of levels to investigate the reflective abilities displayed in the journals of student teachers (Van Manen, 1977; Moon, 1999a). Van Manen's levels are:

- Level 1 – Technical rationality: effective application of technical knowledge in order to reach known outcomes.
- Level 2 – Practical rationality: teachers' ability to deal with practical actions where there are multiple factors in operation. There is an ability to cope with the confusion and make an assessment of the likely educational consequences.
- Level 3 – In Wedman and Martin's terms, this level of critical rationality 'focused on incorporating consideration of moral and ethical criteria into discourse about practical action. The central question at this level was which educational goals, experiences and activities led toward forms of life that were just and equitable.'

It is interesting that there are again elements in common between this schema and the previous two. In Wedman and Martin's research, the contents of the 44 journals were analysed into thought units (Bales, 1957), and were then attributed to the three levels. All but four of the students demonstrated level 1 reflection; one was at level 2 and several appeared to be in transition between levels 1 and 2. The fact that they were in transition was taken to suggest that there is progressive development through the levels.

'Purpose-made' assessment tools

A 'framework for reflective thinking' as an assessment tool. This framework was developed for a pre-teaching programme that particularly promotes reflective approaches. It was developed in order to assess the effectiveness of the approach (Sparkes-Langer *et al*, 1990; Sparkes-Langer and Colton, 1991). The framework is as follows:

Level 1 – no descriptive language
Level 2 – simple, layperson description
Level 3 – events labelled with appropriate terms
Level 4 – explanation with tradition or personal preference given as the rationale

Level 5 – explanation with principle or theory given as the rationale
Level 6 – explanation with principle/theory and consideration of context factors
Level 7 – explanation with consideration of ethical, moral, political issues

Again this framework, like those previously, provides a hierarchy of increasing complexity of material. In this case the research based on the framework did involve independent coders. Inter-coder reliability was 81 per cent (for matches one or less level different) when the material was based on the ideas given in the framework. Reliability was less (not given) for the journal, 'possibly' because the format did not match the framework. The journal was subsequently modified to match the framework items. The need to alter the journal seems to be a considerable indictment of the framework. An assessment instrument for journal writing or reflective writing would seem to require to be of sufficient generality to cover the diversity of writing that can desirably result from a journal. There are some similarities between this approach and that taken later in this chapter.

Criteria for the recognition of evidence of reflectivity in writing. The work of Hatton and Smith (1995) arose from somewhat more thorough research than many of the studies described earlier. While the work derives from the context of teacher education, the descriptions of reflectiveness in writing are generally applicable. A summary of the framework with quotations from it is provided below:

- Descriptive writing (which is considered not to show evidence of reflection) is a description of events or literature reports. There is no discussion beyond description.
- Descriptive reflection: There is description of events but some justification in relatively descriptive language. The possibility of alternative viewpoints in discussion is accepted. Reflection may be 'based generally on one perspective factor as rationale or, presumably in a more sophisticated form, is based 'on the recognition of multiple factors and perspectives'.
- Dialogic reflection: 'Demonstrates a "stepping back" from the events and actions leading to a different level of mulling about discourse with self and exploring the discourse of events and actions'. Uses the 'qualities of judgements and possible alternatives for explaining and hypothesizing'. The reflection is analytical or integrative, linking factors and perspectives. It may reveal inconsistency 'in attempting to provide rationales and critique'.
- Critical reflection: 'Demonstrates an awareness that actions and events are not only located within and explicable by multiple perspectives, but are located in and influenced by multiple historical and socio-political contexts'.

(Hatton and Smith, 1995)

General comments on schemes of assessment criteria

Throughout these criteria-based assessment schemes, which have been developed in different contexts, there are some obvious similarities in the way that the increasingly sophisticated reflective writing is viewed. The most elementary form of writing in the schemata above is simply descriptive. There are then various ways of describing the involvement of greater complexity in the process, the ability to deal with several views of the same event and the possible conflict in views. Helpfully, Hatton and Smith talk about the increasing ability to 'step back' from the event and view it with a broader perspective. This quality seems to progress towards the most sophisticated form of reflective writing, where there is a demonstration of the understanding of the ethical, historical and socio-political context of the issue.

This sequence of increasingly sophisticated function in reflective writing relates closely to the schema of knowledge constitutive interests developed by Habermas (1971) and described in relation to reflection in Moon (1999a). The sequence of three patterns of knowing represents forms of inquiry that 'guide and shape' human knowledge (Carr and Kemmis, 1986). The implication for journal writing is important. It suggests that the level of functioning of journal writers is a representation of their ability to gain access to different forms of knowing.

An interesting question that emerges concerns the degree to which learners can be coached to write at these different levels. For example, Dart *et al* (1998) used the Hatton and Smith descriptors (above) as an assessment tool in their research on the increase of knowledge from the use of learning journals. Most of their subjects produced writing gauged to be 'descriptive reflection'. If the subjects had been coached in the different degrees of reflectiveness in their writing, would they or could they have functioned at a more sophisticated level, then, perhaps changing the result of the experiment?

The forms of assessment of reflective writing above mostly serve their purpose within the context of their use. They are probably as reliable as any other form of assessment in higher education but there are some remaining questions of their validity if we are unsure what really happens when students write reflectively. Earlier in this book we introduced a map of reflective writing which suggests the elements and events of writing reflectively (Figure 2.1 – Chapter 2). This map was then applied to the process of helping learners to start to write journals (Chapter 7) and it is applied again in this chapter to enable a broad reconsideration of the reflective writing process in the context of assessment. For convenience we reproduce the map in Figure 8.1.

Using the map of reflective writing as a source of assessment indicators

The sections above indicate that assessment of journals is often based on a narrow view of the process. At the extreme it is, for example, what might be called 'physical factors' such as measures of length or frequency of entry. Sometimes it is based on the outcome of the process, such as the use of the SOLO taxonomy. At other times it is based on the quality of the reflective discussion. No approach seems to treat the process of writing journals in the breadth and depth that is suggested by the map of reflective writing (Figure 2.1/8.1). If we relate the map to the schemes for assessing journals earlier in this chapter, many do focus on the reflective thinking element of

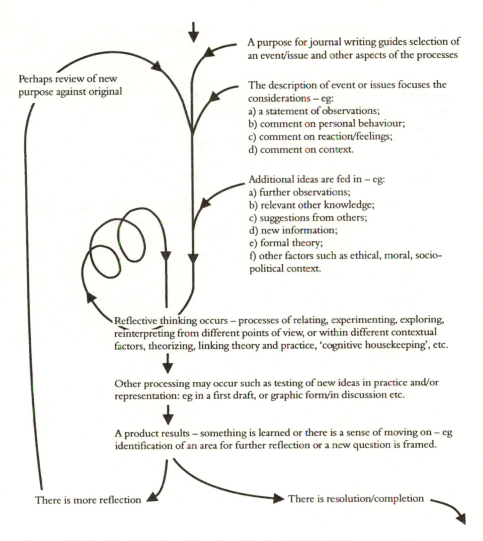

A purpose for journal writing guides selection of an event/issue and other aspects of the processes

Perhaps review of new purpose against original

The description of event or issues focuses the considerations – eg:
a) a statement of observations;
b) comment on personal behaviour;
c) comment on reaction/feelings;
d) comment on context.

Additional ideas are fed in – eg:
a) further observations;
b) relevant other knowledge;
c) suggestions from others;
d) new information;
e) formal theory;
f) other factors such as ethical, moral, socio-political context.

Reflective thinking occurs – processes of relating, experimenting, exploring, reinterpreting from different points of view, or within different contextual factors, theorizing, linking theory and practice, 'cognitive housekeeping', etc.

Other processing may occur such as testing of new ideas in practice and/or representation: eg in a first draft, or graphic form/in discussion etc.

A product results – something is learned or there is a sense of moving on – eg identification of an area for further reflection or a new question is framed.

There is more reflection

There is resolution/completion

Figure 8.1 *A map of reflective writing (reproduction of Figure 2.1)*

writing. However, it is interesting to note that they often start with 'description' of the event. On the map, **description of the event or issue** is a separate event that it is reasonable to assume is present – implicitly or explicitly – if one is to reflect. On that basis, 'description' might be better described as 'no reflective thinking'. It is also noticeable that none of the assessment schemes seem to require the involvement of **additional ideas** – as is depicted on the map.

Because the map attempts to cover the elements involved in journal writing, it provides the basis for development of a comprehensive list of assessment indicators for reflective writing or writing in a journal. We use the term 'indicators' on the basis that more precise and purpose-designed criteria may be developed from the more crudely worded indicators.

We are not suggesting that every time a learner settles down to write an entry in a journal, all of the elements identified on the map should unfold one after another and should be assessed. We are suggesting, instead, that the tutor may identify some elements that are more important than others for the purpose for which the journal is being used and can ask the learner to demonstrate them. In that way, only some indicators would be brought into play for assessment purposes. For example, if the journal is being used to raise consciousness of the impact of the social setting on education, the tutor may be concerned that social variables are brought into the reflective process (in additional ideas). Another way of using the list of assessment indicators would be to ask learners to develop their own criteria based on the indicators. The assessment criteria thus listed could be used for marking by the learners themselves, their peers or their tutor, or – along Burnard's line (above) – by all three.

The list is treated as a checklist of the evidence of events occurring in reflective writing (presence of description, additional information etc) or a selection of areas for focus may be made and the indicators developed as criteria graded in order to allocate marks. The focus is most likely to rest on the quality of the reflective thinking in the journal, and even from the notes on the map, some hierarchy is evident. For example, 'theorizing' might be seen to be of a higher order of thinking than the reorganization of thoughts in 'cognitive housekeeping', but other hierarchies, such as those mentioned – of Habermas, Van Manen, Perry or Belenky *et al* – could be developed. Another focus might be on the product that results from the process.

The assessment indicators are listed below.

Purpose. The learner demonstrates:

awareness and understanding of the purpose of the journal, using the purpose to guide selection and description of event/issue on which to reflect.

The learner identifies:

her own purpose for the journal or journal entry.

The description of an event or issue:

is present.

The description:

provides an adequate focus for further reflection.

It includes:

- a statement of observations;
- comment on personal behaviour;
- comment on reaction/feelings;
- comment on context.

Additional ideas:

are present.

The learner demonstrates:

- the introduction of (any) additional ideas to the description;
- the addition of:
  - further observations;
  - relevant other knowledge, experience, feelings, intuitions;
  - suggestions from others;
  - new information;
  - formal theory;
  - other factors such as ethical, moral, socio-political context.

Reflective thinking:

is present.

The learner demonstrates:

- the ability to work with unstructured material;
- the linking of theory and practice;
- the viewing of an issue/event from different points of view;
- the ability to 'step back' from a situation;
- metacognitive processes;
- 'cognitive housekeeping';
- application of theoretical ideas;
- considerations of alternative interpretations;
- etc.

Other processing. There is evidence of other processing – eg

- new ideas are tested in practice;
- new ideas are represented, for example, in a first draft or graphic form etc and there is evidence of review and revision in a later copy.

A product results. The is a statement of:

- either something that has been learned or solved that relates to the purpose or the problematic nature of the description; or
- there is a sense of moving on. For example, there is identification of a new area for further reflection or a new question is framed.

We reiterate the important point that assessment of reflective writing or the journal should take account of the purpose for which the journal has been written by referring again to the work of Dart *et al*. This group of researchers demonstrates that the quality of journal writing can be assessed against a number of variables in addition to those considered in the schemes above. For example, they evaluated journals for the quality of information contained, the connections between teaching and learning, the professional development indicated and the metacognitive thinking displayed.

Part IV

Using journals more effectively: journal examples and activities

Chapter 9

Examples of journals

Introduction

To this point, the content of this book has focused on features of journal writing or on the internal content of journals. It has considered the manner in which we learn from journals (Chapter 2), purposes (Chapters 3 and 8), the way in which to set up journal writing (Chapter 7) and assessment. Review of the content of journals has included journals in learning (Chapter 4), professional development (Chapter 5) and personal development (Chapter 6). This part of the book aims to provide some ideas that will enhance any journal writing in general. This chapter, in particular, moves away from the parts of journals to take a look at several examples of whole journals or methods of using journals (see below). The last chapter provides a range of activities that can be used in any journal (Chapter 10).

The journals or journal methods included in this chapter are chosen because they are frequently mentioned in earlier parts of the book, and for reference and interest purposes are worth consideration in greater detail. Alternatively, they are journal formats that have been found to be useful in particular and various contexts. Some are from my own experience. The aim of the chapter is to provide ideas, guidance and the encouragement to get involved in an area of writing in which the possibilities are boundless. We have not included in this chapter journals that are specifically designed to support discipline learning in higher education courses because the better descriptions of these tend to have been included in Chapter 4.

The first two examples represent methods of using journals as well as discussion of journal format. The first (1) is the Intensive Journal of Progoff, to which reference has been made in many parts of this book. The second (2) is a description of a manner of using journals as a support to the learning in training and short courses. This and the following three examples are developments from my own long-term use of journals and represent different manners in which I have found value in journal activities, both personally and with others. The third example (3) describes a form of a journal that has a strong function as an organizer of personal activity as well as a means of support and development of personal learning. The next (4) is also a personal journal – it is the format of journal that has evolved as my own personal development journal over many years of use. Alongside my personal journal, I have recently found immense value in using a project journal (5). The project, in this case, is this book. The last case study (6) is again of a journal to which a number of references have been made in the text. It is a journal that was developed by Morrison (1990, 1996) to accompany learning on a modular postgraduate programme.

1. Progoff's Intensive Journal

Progoff's background is of significance to understanding his development of the Intensive Journal because his orientation influenced the structure of the journal (Progoff, 1975). Progoff, for example, studied under Carl Jung for a time. He was also one of the founders of the Association for Humanistic Psychology but was neither a therapist nor only a psychologist. Kaiser (1981) describes him as a philosopher theologian alongside Buber and Tillich. Similarly to them, Progoff was interested in the meaning that people could make of their lives and the events that confront them. The spiritual element is clear in the books that Progoff wrote about the journal and its processes and in the nature of the workshops that are designed to introduce the journal (Progoff, 1975, 1980). The workshops are described alongside the journal structure in Progoff (1975).

The Intensive Journal consists of 19 sections in which the writer works. Progoff describes this form of the journal as representing: 'An instrument ... capable of drawing together the multiplicity of contents of human life, (and) compressing them into a more manageable space while not losing the quality of movement and change that is their essence'(1975: 21). The structure evolved both from his research work in depth psychology where he was concerned with people's life histories, and from his therapeutic work.

Each section in the Intensive Journal is associated with a particular type of subject matter and/or with particular methods of writing. A number of the methods of working are described in the last chapter (Chapter 10) as activities. Examples of the sections are Daily log (recording of daily events), Dream log (for recording dreams) and Dialogue sections (a number of sections that are related by the use of a dialoguing method). On any occasion writers might start by recording in the daily log section and move from there to work on other aspects of their current experience in different ways in other sections, always cross-referencing the entries. Another time they might start with a section that is associated with a form of activity that generates memories to explore further (Steppingstones – see Chapter 10). There is also a Life history log for material that relates to the writer's previous life story. These descriptions may be specific or they may represent brief memories that have arisen in connection with writing in another part of the journal. Another interesting section is Intersections (see Chapter 10). This relates to 'roads taken and not taken' (1975: 145) – to decision points in life where a decision is made to take one course of action as opposed to another. Progoff suggests that there can be value in examining the decision not taken as there may be matters still of value to learn.

By flowing between the past, present and future and across different sections of the journal, the writer integrates the various elements of his or her life and develops a greater sense of self – 'who I am'. We have mentioned that Progoff's journal has been used effectively with unemployed groups and it has had frequent use in situations of spiritual development or exploration.

Unfortunately, the book that describes the use of the journal is not very accessible, being written in a ponderous and meditative mode to accompany and match the atmosphere of the workshops. Other literature that interprets Progoff's work is a better introduction to the methods, although it loses something of the spiritual nature of the whole experience of attending a workshop and continuing to write in the recommended style. Examples of useful and reasonably comprehensive references to Progoff's work are Rainer (1978), Miller (1979), Kaiser (1981), Cell (1984), Hallberg (1987), Burnham (1987) and Lukinsky (1990), among many others.

2. Using journals to support learning in short courses

The origin of this work was my involvement in professional development in the health service (health promotion). In my role, I was concerned with short training courses, largely for nurses, of one or two days or slightly longer. I was concerned that it was all too easy for participants to sign on and to attend the course – and then to go back to their workplace and do nothing different. The course did not have impact. There might be several reasons for this. The course might have been taught badly, the participant may not have found it relevant, but often I felt that the reason was that the new behaviour suggested in the course was not sufficiently linked into the participant's current behaviour patterns. Back in the workplace, with work piled up from the day or two on the course, it was easier for the participant to put the ideas on one side ('for when I have more time to think about it all') and to carry on with old patterns. It became evident that this was a pattern that was true for many courses.

One approach to increasing the impact of short courses is to specify the improvement of practice in terms of anticipated learning outcomes, instead of being concerned only with the learning that should be achieved in the training period. Developing from this is the need to embed the ideas by developing plenty of time for reflection in the period of the course. However, just reflecting on the content of the course is not sufficient. There needs to be consideration of how the new ideas fit into the current practice and can result in changed or improved practice. It is a process that needs imagination and reflection – and still this is not all. The knowledge that professionals such as nurses and teachers have of their practice tends to be tacit and often not readily expressed or modified without some encouragement (Schön, 1983).

On a short course there is little time or opportunity for participants to learn new ideas and go through these various stages of embedding the ideas into their understanding of their practice. This is where journals are useful – even for one-day courses. I have found the following framework to be useful as a structure that can underpin the reflective writing that goes into a journal and it will probably guide the sequence of a course as well. It is divided into four phases:

- Phase 1: An awareness of current practice with regard to the subject matter of the course is developed.
- Phase 2: The content of the new learning is clarified and related to the current understandings.
- Phase 3: The new learning is considered in relationship to the current practice.
- Phase 4: There is anticipation and imagination of the nature of the changed/improved practice. It will be based on the question 'What will you do that is different tomorrow?'.

Journal writing that roughly follows this sequence will facilitate the embedding of the new ideas into practice. During the course, there will be periods for reflective activity. These periods may involve pairing off and talking about the material that has just been presented and then making journal entries on the basis of discussion, or they may involve just writing.

It is hard to achieve much change in practice in a day. However, the reflective activity even on a day course can be extended. I nearly always ask participants to do 'prework' before a course. This usually involves a set of up to five questions (around 15 minutes' work) which are designed to develop an appropriate mind-set to the material of the course before the participants arrive, and it can easily incorporate questions about the current work practices. The prework represents the first entries into the journal and I ask for one set of it to be sent to me so that I can integrate it into the course activities.

The extension of a course in the other direction can be achieved by the requirement that participants produce some assignment task or a report in order to be 'signed off' or awarded a course certificate or university credit. The assignment may, for example, be a learning journal recording the process of instituting the change in practice or it might be a piece of writing that requires reference to an ongoing reflective account that relates to the impact of the course.

3. A 'daybook' that supports professional activity and learning

Over the past eight years, I have developed and used a daybook system to support my activity and learning in three different work situations. Most of the work was developmental, somewhat unpredictable and, in some form, involved a multiplicity of networking and meetings with people in different locations or work.

The daybook probably only just qualifies as a form of journal as it is on the edge of being more like a record-keeping system – but there is some learning output. From early on I used an A5 (or roughly half letter size) loose-leaf file for the daybook. I cut and punch my own pages (half A4/letter size) and I made the section dividers. Personalizing even this professional activity book seemed to be important and it is covered in blue leather that helps also with wear and tear. It is constantly with me. The daybook contains the following sections:

- In front of the first section I carry spare paper and unfiled meetings notes (see later).
- 'Records'. This section is a recent addition. At times I have needed to make lists of people I have needed to contact about a particular issue, and in this section, I would, for example, note on the list when I had contacted them and when I had visited them.
- 'To do' – a vital section in terms of organization. The list develops and extends, with items crossed out as they are dealt with. Every so often I rewrite the list afresh. This always brings a sense of greater organization as the expansive list with many crossed-out items condenses back onto one page. I usually have a page of longer-term 'to do's' at the front of this section.
- 'Thoughts'. This is the 'learning' part of the daybook. I 'capture' stray ideas here, think them through on paper, add to them, sometimes lifting them into a more permanent place among other notes or papers. The section may be the home for the initial ideas for a project or the development of notes from a meeting. In spare moments I go through the material that accumulates there.
- 'Contacts and references'. This section is for making a quick note of work contacts, phone numbers, and sometimes references. The material here may be lifted into my diary.
- 'Meeting list'. This and the next section have been crucial to my networking activities. The 'meeting list' section contains a list of all meetings that I attend and phone calls where there is information that I need to keep. The notes of the meetings are filed in the next section ('Meetings'). The Meeting List provides a number for the meeting, the name of the person or group that I met, and sometimes the location of the meeting.
- 'Meetings'. Here are filed the notes of meetings. They have been written on a home-made A5, or roughly half letter size, clip board. Each page is numbered (theoretically in red) with the same reference number that relates to the previous section. At one time I rewrote all of the notes after meetings. Now I do that only for more complex or important notes. This section tends to fill up and then I remove notes to store elsewhere – usually bound with a treasury tag – but with dates and numbers still easy to locate from the 'meeting list'.

4. Evolving a format for a personal journal

In Chapter 1 I introduced my own journal writing activity as a part of the entrée to this book. It does have that role and I would probably not be writing this book were it not for that personal enthusiasm. In this section I will be more objective about my own experiences in considering how they have led me to design and redesign formats for journals. Such a process does not seem unusual among journal writers. Rainer (1978) and Grumet (1990) are among others who describe similar evolutions.

I go back now to the experience of learning to use Progoff's Intensive Journal, and the significance of that for my journal writing habit. For a while I wrote in most of the 19 sections of the journal, particularly while I was able to get to the series of associated workshops. Then, as with many of us who started, the ability to sustain the effort overcame my enthusiasm and the maintained sections tailed off towards a daily recording in the daily log, period and dream log recording and work in other sections on occasions. I also rapidly ran out of space in the A4/letter-sized file which was provided at the workshop and found that A5 (or roughly half letter size) pages were much more convenient and portable. I made two new sets of section dividers. One set went into a small personalized file for 'every day' journal writing and once a year or so, I would move the accumulation of journal material into a larger file. I found that the fat A5 files in which weekly instalments of recipes or gardening hints were to be placed provided a useful location for the journal material. This maintained my daily journal at a reasonably portable size.

I have maintained a journal regularly in this way, for many years. This has meant a bulging section for the daily log, entries in the period log and slim fillings for one or two other sections and little elsewhere. I particularly enjoy maintaining the period log, looking back over a period of time and considering it as a distinctive whole, with images and feelings that are associated with it but that are different from those of another period. I find it intriguing to sense when a period of my life is coming to an end and when, suddenly sometimes, a new period has begun. I also put into this section a copy of the letter I write each Christmas to friends, as this is form of period log whose timing is enforced by the pattern of the year. During these years I would write my journal at the end of the day. It seemed to take on the role of a closing down of the day, and in writing, I would feel easy and settled.

Most of the content of my journal has always concerned my emotional life, with relatively little writing concerning description of events. This changed, however, when I was travelling. Then I would want to be descriptive and also I would not want to carry the A5 file (often I would have a backpack). I have several times, therefore, punched a number of sheets of paper and two pieces of stiff board, sandwiched the paper between the boards and used treasury tags to hold it all together. As a light travel journal, such arrangements have worked well and the paper has been re-filed with my normal journal on return.

Perhaps it was the stirring of thought about journals caused by the emerging notion of this book that gave rise to the next stage of evolution in which my habit is located at the present time. I decided that just writing at the end of the day, as a kind of summary activity, was not satisfactory any longer. I wanted to be able to write notes, descriptions of events, to think on the paper of my journal at any time. This posed problems of portability. My A5 file could not be carried easily because A5 would not fit into a convenient size of handbag. I did not want to reduce the paper size because I would have felt constrained by a very small page on which to write. I could have moved on to using a pocket organizer. I therefore decided to fold in half the A5 paper (to A6, or roughly quarter letter size) and protect it with two slightly larger than A6 boards that are jointed in the middle so that they fold over the folded paper (Figure 9.1). Treasury tags through holes in the paper and boards hold it all together.

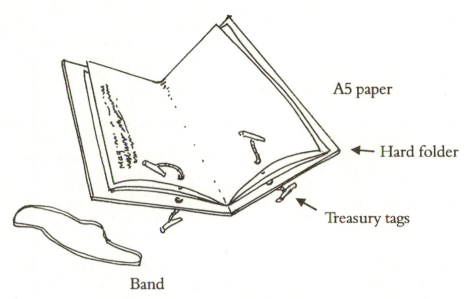

A5 paper

← Hard folder

Treasury tags

Band

Figure 9.1 *A portable A5, or roughly half letter size, journal*

As with the daybook (5), personalizing a journal seems to be important. Mine is covered with suede and I have a red band around it to prevent the paper from 'flopping out'. There are only a few pages in the portable journal and when one is written on both sides, I transfer it into the old A5 file.

This arrangement has proved to be relatively satisfactory. I would prefer to write on a larger page than folded A5, but portability seems to be more important at present. However, in making this change of format, I confronted another issue. How would I deal with all the sections of the Intensive Journal, which I did still occasionally use? It was hard to change a habit of some 20 years, but I admitted to myself that I was not using the sections on a regular enough basis to maintain all the divisions and I needed to make the whole thing simpler. I have arrived at a format of two sections only. One is the daily log. The other is a section for anything else – 'workings' I call it. It is a section for anything other than daily entry material – for dreams, for stray thoughts, journal activities (Chapter 10), systematic 'thinking through' or for period log entries. These entries are dated and given a title and there is a cross-reference into the daily log section. In many ways, this system is relatively similar to that of Rainer with her 'diary tools' but both do rely on a working knowledge of a range of techniques that can be called into use when there is need or there is time to explore. There are plenty of examples of these in Chapter 10.

5. A project journal

The development of a project journal has, perhaps, been one of the greatest areas of personal learning for me in the process of writing this book and it is certainly an activity I would undertake with any form of project in the future. The origins were in notes about learning journals that began to accumulate around the time that the publishing proposal was submitted. The notes were on A5 (or roughly half letter size) paper for portability and ring bound. Fairly soon after that I slotted in dividers for each proposed chapter heading so that stray thoughts could be entered in an appropriate 'home'. Sometimes I would focus on a particular chapter and do a personal 'brainstorm', often during some form of exercise session at the end of an evening of writing. This meant that the notes for the chapters built up and the chapter-headed sections became the location also for writing planning notes and listing the literature to which I wanted to refer.

In terms of the project notebook becoming a 'true' learning journal, the crucial decision was to add a section for dated entries of reflection on the progress of the project. This took off. I did not record in the 'journal section' every day, but it became the location for comments and for 'thinking on paper' about the progress of the book. Miller (1979) talks about the value of journals in enhancement of creativity because the passage of the thoughts is recorded so that the mind is clear to move on to other thoughts, while a record of the 'train' of thinking is retained. My experience is in accordance with her comment.

I review the process of writing through the 'eye' of the journal:

- The first entries seem to be furnishing a background to the potential book, locating it in a history of interests in journal writing and reflection and identifying my feelings about writing another book so soon after the last.
- There are several recordings about library searches, looking for information on the World Wide Web, and some enthusiastic writing about particular texts such as that of Rainer (1978) – 'Reading Rainer's book is wonderful. I keep making discoveries about me and why I write a journal.'
- Soon after that I made some entries about the reorganization of my personal journal into a more portable format (see (4) above). There is a drawing of how I wanted it to look.
- There is an entry about how I began to think about categorizing the heap of photocopied papers and extracts that had accumulated. I decided to number them and list their names against the numbers as another section in the journal. This proved to be enormously useful.
- Christmas came and went and I recorded that there was a building sense of urgency to write. In these entries there are the deliberations about the sequence in which to write. It was Chapter 8, on the assessment of reflection, that I decided to write first. It gave me something useful to discuss with others who were interested in journals from early on.
- In later entries there are sequences of ideas, the decision making about chapter lengths in relation to the book length, a few comments about progress in writing

– but it tails off. There is a comment that the further I move into the book itself, the less I seem to need to write the journal. There is a growing sense of anticipation of reaching the end and of noting the date on which the book is finished – but maybe recording it will not matter then.

Although this is not the first book that I have written, I have learnt a great deal more about the management of information and the whole book-writing process through the process of thinking on paper in one place. It would otherwise have been on a series of scrap sheets consigned to the bin as soon as I had passed through that stage. Using a project journal is certainly a process that I would repeat for another book – one, in fact, that I have begun to repeat for the next book....

6. A journal in a professional development Master's programme (Morrison, 1996)

Various references have been made to Morrison's use of journal writing in earlier chapters (1990, 1996). Morrison's work is interesting because it is rooted in theoretical ideas, promotes personal, professional and academic development and has a particular role in the course that he describes. The journal is employed in the context of a modular Master's degree in education. One of its roles is to support reflective practice over the period of study, 'developing in students, the ability to be self-monitoring, self-directive and professionally autonomous'. This has particular relevance in the potentially fragmented learning environment of a modular programme.

The development of reflective practice in Morrison's work is based on two models of reflection. The first, which he equates with Schön's reflection-in-and-reflection-on practice, concerns short-term matters such as specific events, rather than long-term issues of personal relationship to society (Schön, 1983). The long-term issues for reflection are the subject matter of the second model. The concerns of the second model relate to a person's state in a social setting, issues of power and empowerment with the aim as emancipation. Students are introduced to these models in the context of their journal activities. In terms of the subject matter of the first model, they are asked to reflect in a day-to-day manner on their programme, on their study habits, on their reading, on significant events, decisions, insights and the views that they hold. They are also invited to consider the progression and development in their knowledge, practice, attitudes, understanding and so on. This reflection is supported by banks of questions.

The second model of reflective practice is based on the work of Prawat (1991). Students are invited to consider developments in the functioning that underlies personal power – their 'voice', their view of themselves in their settings and their knowledge of and relationships to the power in those settings.

The journals are not themselves assessed. However, as we have indicated previously (Chapter 8), an assignment is based directly on the content of the journal, which effectively forces students to reread and learn more from their writing.

Chapter 10

Activities to enhance learning from journals

Introduction

Activities such as are suggested in this chapter may be part of the structure of a journal or they may be offered to learners to use – if they wish. They are offered somewhat in the same spirit as the 'tools' offered by Rainer (1978) (Chapter 6), though there are many more on offer here. Learners will often find activities or exercises particularly helpful when they first start to write because the nature of an activity may lead them into reflecting when they are not initially confident in this form of working. Those who are using journals independently for personal development may wish, on occasions, to use an activity in order to vary their patterns of reflection. Activities can 'trip' writers into useful confrontations with issues that they have consciously avoided in free writing. In this sense, activities can deepen reflective activity. While 'writing' is the word mostly used, drawings that display meaning in a different manner can provide unanticipated learning or surprise.

The activities are organized in eight groups on the basis of broad similarity, but many could fit into other sections. In order to provide an accessible resource for those using journals, we have sometimes repeated journal activities in this chapter from earlier in the book.

Activities associated with encouraging reflective writing

Take a theme

Schneider and Killick (1998) describe how the wife of the aviator, Lindbergh, would wander along the seashore and find a shell each day. She would describe the shell and, from her description, would move into her journal entry. An object can focus attention and provide a starting point. It can provide a sense of continuity, and a metaphor (see later).

Use questions

A number of examples of journal writing systems have been introduced in this book where questions have been used to generate reflection. Sometimes the questions have been developed into a framework (eg Johns, 1994) which takes learners through a sequence of reflecting according to the requirements of the programme. Johns, for example, uses questions to guide reflection on an event or action involving the writer, in this case in nursing practice, and similarly Smyth's framework (1989) encourages reflection ultimately on power and politics of self in a social setting. Questions help learners to get started in reflecting or to deepen their reflection. They may be used in the early stages of journal writing and learners encouraged to be self-guided when they are ready. A well-posed question can lead reluctant writers into reflective activity before they realize that they are fulfilling the requirement of journal writing. A useful and wide-ranging question for students on a course is: 'At this moment, how are you feeling about being a (discipline/subject) student?' (Hahnemann, 1986). Paul (1990) and Morgan and Saxon (1991) also provide some useful principles for questioning.

Generate questions

There is, of course, no reason why learners should not learn to ask questions of each other or of themselves. This example is from Hahnemann (1986). Before a class discussion on a topic, students are asked to write questions about the topic in their journals. A discussion is then held on the topic, and presumably students might be asked to reflect on the discussion afterwards.

Lists

An activity described by Progoff (1975) is particularly useful for generating material on which to reflect and write, or for exploring an idea. The exercise is called 'Steppingstones' and here it is described in a minimal form. On a particular topic learners are asked to list around seven experiences of the topic in strict chronological order. It is likely that when they are getting towards the end of the list, other thoughts that belong previously in the sequence will arise. These are used in a second list, and again are located in chronological sequence. A series of lists can be generated that usually surprise the learner in their extent, particularly where the initial reaction of the learner is 'I don't remember much about that'. The listing is facilitated if, during the activity, each participant is asked to make a general statement to the other participants about his or her list and how he or she is viewing the topic, and to mention, in brief, one memory that has arisen. This can spur new ranges of memories in others. The topic for Steppingstones can be an object, an idea, a place, the relationship with a person – there are no limits. Rainer (1978) also refers to the use of lists in journals.

Concept mapping or graphic representations of ideas

The material in a journal does not need to be written. Graphic techniques can generate new ways of seeing things that can then be explored further in writing. A concept map encapsulates an idea and the themes radiate from the main idea and subdivide hierarchically (Moon, 1999a). Buzan (1993) and Deshler (1990) elaborate on this. The technique can be used individually or in small groups to generate thought that can then be the subject of writing. Several people can make separate maps on a topic and then can compare them. This can demonstrate conceptual differences that underpin learning. Hadwin and Winne (1996) review studies of concept mapping as a study strategy *per se*.

Free writing

In 1973, Elbow suggested that a good means of freeing the style and thoughts of writers is to let writing free-flow on a topic – not correcting or criticizing it for a period of time (eg 10 minutes). He describes this process of writing as being like a sea voyage. 'For the sea voyage you are trying to lose sight of land – the place you began…. In coming to a new land you develop a new conception of what you are writing about.'

Elbow's idea was incorporated into a technique called 'teacher journal' by Yinger (1985). Learners write in 'free-flow' for around 10 minutes. If they run out of ideas, they are asked to write about how it feels to have run out of ideas. They then reread and reflect on what they have written, then dialogue with another about the experience in a manner similar to co-counselling (see later). It would seem appropriate then to ask them to reflect and write again.

'Take a sentence'

Hahnemann (1986) asks her students to 'take one sentence from your readings that sparked your interest and write on its meaning'.

Reflecting on own writing

It may be useful to distinguish between reflection on the learning that emerges from one's writing, reflection on the process of writing in a journal and using a reread to generate ideas for further reflection. In more formal terms, any of these outcomes can be encouraged by use of a double entry technique where one side of the page is for descriptive writing and the other is for further reflections on that writing.

Show learners your journal (as their teacher), or the successful journals of others

Sharing the content of journals has a general facilitatory effect on writing. Those new to journal writing may welcome the opportunity to look at journals that have been written for a while. They may be shown by the writers who can give peer support, or they may be shown anonymous journals that exemplify good practice.

Learning about and managing one's own behaviour

Studying aspects of one's own behaviour

Joanna Field (1951) wanted to learn more about her own behaviour. A simple example of the manner in which she learned more was to note at the end of each day what had made her happy – a moment, a person, an object. In a similar way, other life experiences can provide a focus for writing – but the regular feature of Field's recording allows an observation of pattern over a period of time. Regular recording of other experiences is suggested by Miller (1979). They might be peak experiences and observations of hang-ups.

Period log

This is, again, one of Progoff's journal activities, which is mentioned in the example in Chapter 9. It is based on an observation that one's life does not simply flow in a smooth and unchanging path, but, over periods of time, has one theme or dominant feeling which then changes. The period log records the characteristics of a period of time. Most frequently it will be the period of time most recent to the present, and the period will have stretch back as far as the dominant theme or feeling stretches back. From personal experience, this can be from a few days to a few months, but for myself, it has been no longer than this. The period log gives a sense of the flow of life and it sets a useful context for the other aspects of journal writing, whether they are for personal or formal educational reasons.

Sub-personalities

While the last activity provided a longitudinal view of life, in a sense this one provides a cross-section. Miller (1979) suggests that journal writing is a useful means of exploring and identifying one's sub-personalities, perhaps providing them with names and noting when they arise. Hunt (1987) also considers the study of sub-personalities. He suggests a method of exploration by use of personally guided imagery.

Dialogues

A number of writers mention the use of dialogues, but Progoff's approach is more sophisticated. Dialogues are like scripts for a play in which the writer 'converses' with another. The other might be a person, a part of oneself, a spiritual leader or mentor, an object, an event, a project... anything or anyone with whom there is 'work' to be done. A helpful example might be some task that one cannot get around to. The dialogue could then explore the blocks. The writing often starts with a greeting and a statement of the problem. The technique is simply to write for oneself and wait 'to see' what the other will say back, recording it then, uncritically.

In the context of this section, dialogues may be with oneself or with parts of oneself, or, perhaps, with a mentor or real or imaginary spiritual guide.

Haiku

Haiku is a three-line poetic form with 17 syllables with five, seven and five on respective lines. Hunt (1987) suggests that the method of condensing characteristics of oneself or one's behaviour into such form is a useful method of self-exploration.

Recording of activity

This exercise returns to more concrete activity, but it produces valuable data for further reflection. The exercise consists of logging one's behaviour or thoughts at regular spaces of time, using an alarm to mark the time. A particularly useful version of this activity for generating discussion if several people have pursued it, is to record one's thoughts periodically thoughout a lecture or class.

Currere

This is technique that is mentioned by Pinar (1975) and several writers who interpret Pinar's work (eg Grumet, 1987; Miller, 1987). Pinar originally developed the exercise in the context of work on the nature of the curriculum in schools, but it has potential for other situations. In essence, the same topic for reflection is related initially in the present, and then with reference to its past, and a third section of writing anticipates the future. Grumet suggests that 'multiple accounts splinter the dogmatism of a single tale. If they undermine the authority of the teller, they also free her from being captured by the reflection provided in a single narrative.'

Autobiographical writing

There are many references to autobiographical writing in relation to journals and in other 'one-off' accounts, particularly in the teacher education literature. The development of autobiography can be a focus of attention in journal writing, and rather than consist just of memories, can utilize activities such as those that are described in these chapters, such as currere, steppingstones, dialogues and so on.

Rehearsal

A helpful means of managing difficult or anxiety-provoking events such as conflict with another, examinations or driving tests is to rehearse them in advance. While they can be rehearsed in imagination, greater focus may be obtained by writing them out. This might take the course of a dialogue or an account of the anticipated event with the writers seeing themselves successfully managing the situation. Going through the account several times and thinking about it is likely to facilitate the eventual enactment of the event for the writer.

Writing letters that are not to be sent

Again, several writers mention this technique (eg, Rainer, 1978; Cooper, 1991). Like rehearsal, above, this is a method that can help with the management of personal behaviour. This might be particularly the case if the content is cathartic in nature.

Decisions taken and the ideas not followed

Progoff (1975) calls this work 'intersections'. The journal work reviews a decision that has already been made. Decisions imply the taking of one path in life and the rejection of another or others. Progoff suggests that sometimes there is still 'energy' left in the path(s) not taken and the course that events might have taken can be worthy of exploration.

Metacognitive activities

Reflect on the act of journal writing

Asking learners to reflect on the act of journal writing can be useful in the manner that any act of metacognition appears to facilitate learning. It can be useful also as a means of unblocking writing if learners say that they do not know what to write – or it can be used as a 'filler' activity if there is a set period for journal writing.

Self-assessment of own learning journal

If journals are to be assessed in a formal learning situation, asking learners to assess their own journals is another means of encouraging reflection on the act of writing a journal. The value of the exercise will be increased greatly if the development of assessment criteria is a collaborative activity between tutors and learners.

Learners choose their own style of reflective writing

Setting a journal writing task for learners is not always easy. There are many reasons that learners may find for arguing against the task. If there are difficulties, it may be worth turning the task initially into one of designing a format for ongoing recording and reflection that the learners then maintain (Stephani, 1999). The task may involve thought about the aims and purpose and outcomes of the writing – and the work may not, in the end, be called a journal.

Observations of personal learning through language

Parker and Goodkin (1987) describe a method of focusing on the manner in which the contribution of personal language to learning is explored by teaching students. They are asked to devote one journal entry per week to a description of an occasion when they have used language to learn something on their course. At the end of the year, they select four or five of these entries and write a short 'informal' paper on 'what they think they have learned about thinking and learning from this process' (Parker and Goodkin, 1987: 48).

Questions that focus on personal experiences of learning

An easy way to help learners to reflect on their own processes is to provide sets of questions that lead them towards reflection. The following set is an example:

- What are the characteristics of an interested and motivated learner?
- What are the characteristics of a non-motivated learner?
- Where do you stand? How do you fit these models?
- When have you been really involved in learning something?
- When have you found learning really difficult?
- What does the difference tell you about yourself?

The learners could decide their own questions or develop similar questions for each other.

Reflection on the process and results of a study skills questionnaire

The use of a study skills questionnaire can provide useful material for metacognitive reflection.

Learning in a class

A lecture or class is recorded. Elements of the material are played back to learners and they are asked to record what was in their minds at the time. The reports may be about the learning process or the content of the material. The outcome for a whole class may yield interesting material for teacher and students about the processes of teaching and learning.

Reflection on an interesting aspect of learning

Learners are asked to go over lecture notes or material from reading and mark the part that is of most interest to them and write about the reasons for that interest.

Consulting inner wisdom

A dialogue technique (see above) is set up between the learner and a 'wisdom figure'. The figure may be an imagined real person (a mentor) or a completely imaginary person or figure. The dialogue is about the writer's methods of study and learning, with advice being offered. This is similar to an example given by Cowan (1998b: 68–69).

Non-verbal methods for working in a journal

Draw an image

Progoff uses the drawing of images to facilitate reflection or to summarize a session of reflection. The image may be meaningful like a metaphor, or a graphic construction from the mind of the learner. Similar to this is to ask learners to summarize a lecture or area of knowledge, or a project, in an image in their journals. There may be writing to accompany the image. A variation on this is to engage in free drawing (as Milner, 1957).

The road map of life

This may be a useful activity with which to introduce journal writing. The passage through life is depicted as a road over a map, like a route. The 'going' may be easy and comfortable (perhaps through beautiful countryside) or rough and bumpy (through steep mountains). There may equally be dark or light, open or closed areas of life. The means of depiction are unlimited. The exercise is probably better done initially on a large piece of paper which may be reduced to fit into a journal, or which is treated as a resource to inspire writing. Like many activities, the map drawn on one day may be completely different on the next day – and the difference probably says something about the occasion of the activity. I did this exercise in the context of educational work with prisoners. While for most people the lines fade through the present into the future, the line for some of the prisoners came to an abrupt halt at the moment of their sentencing.

Holly (1991) suggests a similar activity, which she calls 'timelines', in which life is divided up into sections along a line (eg young childhood, adolescence etc). Key words that relate to the sections and further exploration by way of photographs and other artefacts may be consulted in order to clarify the events.

Dreams

Recording dreams may help to elucidate concerns or issues in life or learning. There are many different books on the interpretation of dreams on the market – and many different methods of interpretation (eg Shohet, 1985). From personal experience, one of the most interesting is the Gestalt method in which an imaginary account of its role in the dream is written for each element of the dream (objects, abstract ideas and places as well as people). When worked out in this way, some elements of a dream may seem to be more significant to the dreamer's current concerns.

Twilight imagery

From personal experience and despite what dream books tell us, dreams cannot always be relied on to appear. Twilight imagery is a term developed by Progoff for the imagery that can spontaneously appear in a relaxed state which Progoff describes to be 'between waking and sleeping' (1975: 77). The imagery is, he suggests, representational or symbolic. The significance of images is that 'we do not consciously or deliberately put these perceptions there. We, ourselves, do not determine what they shall be' (1975: 78). They do, however, seem to be encouraged to flow if we take interest in observing them and recording them. In the section on journals to support creativity (Chapter 6), I described the appearance of a 'bear-mouse' creature in my twilight imagery, and its importance to me.

Rainer suggests another version of twilight imagery. She suggests that the writer starts with an image, relaxes and 'watches' to see what happens.

Draw yourself or a project as a tree

A tree can be tall, strong, twisted, leafy, shady, growing in fertile or arid soil.... There are many words that allow human characteristics to be projected onto the image of a tree and the exercise of projection can generate a useful summary and facilitate unexpected learning.

Working with others on journal activities

In this section, we assume that the material is worked on in pairs or groups. The material may have arisen either from journals or as an outcome of the group/paired work.

Co-counselling

The model of co-counselling is based on the work of Jakins (1970) and Evison and Horobin (1983), and both of these manuals contain activities within co-counselling. Co-counselling is a situation in which usually two participants work together in such a way that first one is listener/counsellor and the other talks, and then for the same length of time the situation is reversed. The 'talker' 'owns' the time, using it to explore an issue of his or her choice or one allocated in a formal situation. The talker may or may not want the listener to ask helpful questions or facilitate the process. Within the context of journal writing, it is likely that the issue will be one that has arisen in the writing process. After the session, the new learning can be recorded.

Critical friends

The system of 'critical friends' is similar to co-counselling, although it may not need to occur in pairs. The difference is in the role of the listener who more actively prompts the talker in the manner in which he or she explores the issue in hand, asking questions that promote deeper reflection, and prevent avoidance of difficult issues.

Joint work on autobiographical material

This is a manner in which learners can help each other to write autobiographical material. One of a pair talks about his or her autobiography and the other prompts, questions and comments in order to work towards 'truths' and material that is useful to the present. The talker writes up the session in draft, and shows it the other who may question further. They work together to form material that is as accurate and helpful to present agendas as possible.

Development of concept maps

Several learners develop concept maps (see earlier) on a topic that they have chosen or that has been given. They then share their maps and discuss the differences in perception of the topic. This is a means of emphasizing the differences in perceptions of the same activity or concept.

Dialogue journals

The literature on dialogue journals dates back a number of years. Early examples tend to emanate from primary school classrooms where pupils were asked to write comments about their classroom activities (thoughts, feelings, observations,...) to which the teacher then individually responded. Subsequent examples involved lecturers and students (Staton, 1988) or students working together, or researchers working in collaborative inquiry (eg Roderick and Berman, 1984). Examples of literature on dialogue journals are given in Staton *et al* (1988). The disadvantage of such a method can often be the time it takes for transmission and response, and modern versions of e-mail discussions can overcome this.

Activities in journals used to support other learning

Improving the learning from creative processes

There are many situations in formal education where a physical object is the outcome of work and the object itself is the subject of assessment. Not only is the process of learning to create the object neglected in assessment terms, but there is a loss of opportunity to reflect on and during the process and to learn from this (Davies, 1998). Journals can play a valuable part in the creative process either to enable assessment to be made of the process, or to enhance learning.

Use journals to enhance learning within the class

There are many ways in which journal writing can enhance classroom learning, both by consolidating and demanding active learning and by providing a change of pace. Some of the suggestions below come from an extract on the World Wide Web of work edited by Jacobson (www):

- A question is displayed for learners when they come into the class. They spend five minutes on it in their journals. The question might initiate thinking about the subject matter of the session.
- There is time for learners to write a summary of a class at the end of the class – or to note issues, or the most significant factors that they have learned (etc).
- Learners are given a break during a lecture to write a response to a question, to note issues that they least understand, to summarize or develop thoughts.
- A similar break is posited in a discussion session or a seminar.

Journals accompany problem solving

Perhaps one of the most useful observations about the use of journals is that writing about the solving of a problem improves the process of problem solving (Jacobson, www; Selfe and Arbabi, 1986; Cowan, 1998b; and others). Learners write or talk about their processes of problem solving rather than following the process 'in their heads'. They seem better able to solve the problem at hand and to learn the process for a later problem.

'Quickthink'

Quickthink is a term coined for situations in which thought-provoking and open-ended questions are given to small groups of learners about a topical subject – one that has just been taught or is about to be introduced. The groups have a short time in which to develop a response, and afterwards the result or useful ideas are written in brief, individually in journals.

Relate theory and practice

A number of writers (eg Hettich, 1976; Wagenaar, 1984; Fulwiler, 1986) use journals with their students to encourage the making of connections between the classroom theory and practical and real-world situations. They ask them to seek out examples of the classroom ideas in everyday life.

Taking a wider picture on field-notes

Field-notes can be strictly scientific only or they can be a means of recording personal feelings along with the observations. This seems to enable learners to 'see' and understand better the subject of their observation (Fulwiler, 1986).

'What if?' questions

These may be part of a 'quickthink' session (above) or an activity alone. 'What if?' questions stretch thought and imagination into areas not normally encountered.

Select areas of confusion

Learners are encouraged to seek out and explore areas of work in which they are confused or uncertain. An atmosphere of trust enables learners to admit their difficulties (Mayher, Lester and Pradl, 1983).

Activities to support reflective practice

A means of learning to reflect on practice

Neary (1998) introduces the notion of reflection on practice to groups of students early in their course by asking them to give a short and relevant presentation and to write a reflective account of their performance in their journals.

Relating one's own learning to that of others

Exploring one's own attitudes towards something or exploring one's processes of performing in some way can be reflectively compared with observations of the equivalent in others. Subject matter might be one's attitude towards authority in a particular and relevant situation.

Critical incident analysis

Critical incident analysis is often seen as a technique on its own that encourages reflective practice but within the context of a journal it is also a useful activity (Ghaye and Lillyman, 1997). A critical incident itself can be just an ordinary incident or one about which there is a special characteristic. In effect it is an incident that is selected for analysis with the expectation that learning from experience will result. The incident is described and then subjected to 'why questions' and other forms of deeper analysis in order to get at the unquestioned aspects of the event and in order to learn from them.

Situations in practice

Learners write about a situation that went well and one that went badly during the day/week. Adding two dimensions to writing with an element of contrast sets up a tension and begs questions on which to bring reflection to bear.

Portraits

Working out relationships with others plays a large part in most practice situations. Rainer (1978) suggests the development of 'portraits' as an activity that enables the writer to gain a picture of another that is separated from the other's role in relation to the writer. Sometimes there is dislike for the person because he or she has something that is a problem similar to one within the writer him/herself. Issues that concern the relationship with others can be seen in a more objective light. The portrait is simply a written description of the person, but not the relationship.

Activities to deepen reflection and the learning from reflective processes

Metaphor

Many of the activities already mentioned involve the use of metaphor directly or indirectly. Richardson (1994) indicates how we tend to perpetuate 'worn out metaphors' in writing. An example is the notion of theory as a building. She suggests that we should try considering theory as tapestry or illness, and then notice the difference it makes to our perception. One way of working with metaphor in a journal is to highlight metaphors that we do use and examine in further entries how they affect the manner in which we view the matter. A progression from that stage is to try allocating new metaphors and determine the effect on perceptions.

Another use of metaphor is illustrated in part in a paper by Reid and Leigh (1998). As a means of assessment of an undergraduate module, students were asked to develop a three-dimensional image as a means of promoting reflection on their learning about organizations. The step beyond the construction that makes this a good journal activity is the reflection on how the construction relates to the learning.

Altered points of view

The same event perceived by different people or from the viewpoint of different life stages of the same person (Rainer, 1978) or by sub-personalities (see above) can seem very different. By enacting the different viewpoints about an indentified issue in the form of imaginary dialogues, it may be possible to attain a deeper and broader understanding of it. Weil (1996), for example, describes how her research on educational experiences was enriched considerably through her 'giving voice' to the different elements of her role as a researcher.

SWOT analysis

In some ways the use of a SWOT analysis is similar to the activity above in focusing on different groupings of factors that are a part of the same whole. A SWOT analysis is a review in terms first of strengths, then of weaknesses, then of the opportunities and lastly of threats to the possibility of change. The review might focus on a person and his or her capacities, an event, a project, a situation, a system – anything. A reflective overview of the analysis may demonstrate some surprises.

Repertory grid

The repertory grid is based on the work of Kelly (1955). Kelly's thesis is that people endeavour to make meaning from the elements of their environment in order to gain control over their lives. As humans, we develop a representational model of the world as a means of organization and the model is unique to an individual because it represents the sense he or she has made. The repertory grid technique elicits the meanings that we construct. In a very simple form it produces interesting data about the way in which we see the world. If the subject matter is the characteristics of people, three people are identified. On the basis of some characteristic, two are identified as similar and one different. The process is repeated with another three people and again a characteristic is identified that distinguishes two from one of them. The characteristics that have been selected represent elements of the construct of personhood for that individual. Eventually the selected characteristics will be repeated and this indicates that the extent of the construct is being reached. The repertory grid can be used for anything, not just people.

Multiple layers of reflection

This activity is an extension of the idea of double entry journals where initial descriptive writing is subjected to reflection at a later stage, with the reflective writing usually written in a column alongside the description, or on the opposite page. Multiple layer reflection is where there is another and perhaps yet another review of the initial description and its initial reflection, perhaps taking in increasingly broad ranges of entries and seeking patterns.

References

Allport, G (1942) *The Use of Personal Documents in Psychological Science*, New York, Social Science Research Council

Ambrose, J (1987) Music journals, in *The Journal Book*, ed T Fulwiler, Heinemann, Portsmouth, NH

Anbar (www) Learning to learn software, Session 5 – The learning log, http://www.anbar.co.uk/courseware/mba/121-005.htm

Anderson, W (1982) The use of journals in a human sexuality course, *Teaching of Psychology*, **9**, pp 105–07

Ashbury, J, Fletcher, B and Birtwhistle, R (1993) Personal journal writing in a communication course for first year medical students, *Medical Education*, **27**, pp 196–204

Aspinwall, K (1986) Teacher biography: the in-service potential, *Cambridge Journal of Education*, **16** (3), pp 210–15

Bales, R (1957) *Interaction Process Analysis,* Addison-Wesley, Reading, MA

Baltensperger, B (1987) Journals in economic geography, in *The Journal Book*, ed T Fulwiler, Heinemann, Portsmouth, NH

Barnett, R (1997) *Higher Education: a Critical Business*, SRHE/OUP, Buckingham

Belenky, M, Clinchy, B, Goldberger, R and Tarule, J (1986) *Women's Ways of Knowing*, Basic Books, New York

Berthoff, A (1987) Dialectical notebooks and the audit of meaning, in *The Journal Book*, ed T Fulwiler, Heinemann, Portsmouth, NH

Biggs, J and Collis, K (1982) *Evaluating the Quality of Learning*, Academic Press, New York

Bloom, B (1956) *Taxonomy of Educational Objectives,* Longmans-Green, New York

Bolton, G and Styles, M (1995) There are stories and stories: an autobiographical workshop, in *The Uses of Autobiography*, ed J Swindells, Taylor and Francis, London

Boud, D, Keogh, R and Walker, D (1985) *Reflection: Turning Experience into Learning*, Kogan Page, London

Boud, D and Miller, N, eds (1996) *Working with Experience*, Routledge, London

Bowman, R (1983) The personal student journal. Mirror of the mind, *Contemporary Education*, **55**, pp 25–27

Bridges, W (1980) *Transitions*, Addison-Wesley, Reading, MA

Britton, J (1972) 'Writing to learn and learning to write', in *The Humanity of English,* National Council of Teachers of English, Urbana, IL

Brockbank, A and McGill, I (1998) *Facilitating Reflective Learning in Higher Education*, SRHE/OUP, Buckingham

Brodsky, D and Meagher, E (1987) Journals and political science, in *The Journal Book*, ed T Fulwiler, Heinemann, Portsmouth, NH

Brown, A, Ambruster, B and Baker, L (1986) The role of metacognition in reading and studying, in *Reading Comprehension from Research to Practice*, ed J Orananu, Lawrence Erlbaum, Hillsdale, NJ

Bruce, R (www) Strange but true: improve your health through counselling, http://www.cybertowers.com/selfhelp/articles/health/journal.html

Bruner, J (1971) *The Relevance of Education*, W W Norton, New York

Bruner, J (1990) *Acts of Meaning*, Harvard University Press, Cambridge, MA

Bunker, A and Cronin, M (1997) Improving students' academic writing with the use of the word processor, in *Learning Through Teaching*, Proc. 6th Annual Teaching Learning Forum, February, Murdoch University, Australia

Burke, P and Rainbow, B (1998) Compile a portfolio, *THES*, 30 October

Burnard, P (1988) The journal as an assessment and evaluation tool in nurse education, *Nurse Education Today*, **8**, pp 105–07

Burnham, C (1987) Reinvigorating a tradition: the personal development journal, in *The Journal Book*, ed T Fulwiler, Heinemann, Portsmouth, NH

Buzan, T (1993) *The Mind Map Book*, BBC Books, London

Calderhead, J and James, C (1992) Recording student teacher's learning experiences, *J Further and Higher Education*, **16** (1), pp 1–3

Canning, C (1991) What the teachers say about reflection, *Educational Leadership*, March

Carlsmith, C (www) An 'academical notebook', http://minerva.acc.virginia.edu/trc/tcacabk.htm

Carr, W and Kemmis, S (1986) *Becoming Critical*, Falmer Press, London

Cell, E (1984) *Learning to Learn from Experience*, Albany State University of New York Press, New York

Christensen, R (1981) 'Dear diary', a learning tool for adults, *Lifelong Learning in the Adult Years*, October

Clarke, B, James, C and Kelly, J (1996) Reflective practice, reviewing the issues and refocusing the debate, *International Journal of Nursing Studies*, **33** (2), pp 171–80

Cooper, J (1991) Telling our own stories, in *Stories Lives Tell: Narrative and dialogue in education*, ed C Whitehead and N Noddings, Teachers College Press, New York

Cowan, J (1998a) Personal communication

Cowan, J (1998b) *On Becoming An Innovative University Teacher*, SRHE/OUP, Buckingham

Creme, P (1998) *New Forms of Student and Assessment in Social Anthropology: Research through practice at the University of Sussex*, National Network in Teaching and Learning Anthropology FDTL Project 1997–1998

Dart, B, Boulton-Lewis, G, Brownlee, J and McCrindle, A (1998) Change in knowledge of learning and teaching through journal writing, *Research Papers in Education*, **13** (3), pp 291–318

Davies, J (1998) Paper given at *Improving Student Learning* Conference, Brighton

Deshler, D (1990) Conceptual mapping: drawing charts of the mind, in *Fostering Critical Reflection in Adulthood*, ed J Mezirow, Jossey-Bass, San Francisco

Dewey, J (1933) *How We Think*, D C Heath and Co, Boston, MA

Didion, J (1968) *Slouching Towards Bethlehem*, Penguin, Harmondsworth

Dillon, D (1983) Self-discovery through writing personal journals, *Language Arts*, **60** (3), pp 373–79

Dimino, E (1988) Clinical journals: a non-threatening strategy to foster ethical and intellectual development development in nursing students, *Virginia Nurse*, **56** (1), pp 12–14

Eisner, E (1991) Forms of understanding and the future of education, *Educational Researcher*, **22**, pp 5–11

Elbow, P (1973) *Writing Without Teachers*, Oxford University Press, New York

Elbow, P (1981) *Writing with Power: Techniques for Mastering the Writing Process*, Oxford University Press, New York

Elbow, P and Clarke, J (1987) Desert island discourse: the benefits of ignoring audience, in *The Journal Book*, ed T Fulwiler, Heinemann, Portsmouth, NH

Elkins, J (1985) Rites of passage. Law students 'telling their lives', *Journal of Legal Education*, **35**, pp 27–55

Emig, J (1977) Writing as a model of learning, *College Composition and Communication*, **28**, pp 122–28

Entwistle, N (1996) Recent research on student learning and the learning environment, in *The Management of Independent Learning*, ed J Tait and P Knight, SEDA/Kogan Page, London

Eraut, M (1994) *Developing Professional Knowledge and Competence*, Falmer Press, London

Ertmer, P and Newby, T (1996) The expert learner: strategic, self-regulated and reflective, *Instructional Science*, **24**, pp 1–24

Evison, R and Horobin, R (1983) *How to Change Yourself and Your World: a manual of co-counselling*, Co-counselling Phoenix, Sheffield

Fazey, D (1993) Self assessment as a genuine tool for enterprising students: the learning process, *Assessment and Evaluation in Higher Education*, **18** (3), pp 335–50

Field, J (1951) *A Life of One's Own*, Penguin, Harmondsworth

Ficher, C (1990) Student journal writing in marketing courses, *Journal of Marketing Education*, Spring, pp 46–51

Finch, A (www) Designing and using a learner journal for false beginners: self-assessment and organization of learning, http://anu.andong.ac.kr/ afinch/paper3.html

Flavell, J (1987) Speculations about the nature and development of metacognition, in *Metacognition, Motivation and Understanding*, ed F Weinett and R Kluwe, Lawrence Erlbaum, Hillsdale, NJ

Flynn, E (1986) Composing responses to literary texts, in *Writing Across the Disciplines*, ed A Young and T Fulwiler, Boynton/Cook Publishers, Upper Montclair, NJ

Fox, R (1982) The personal log, enriching clinical practice, *Clin. Social. Work Journal*, **10**, pp 104–14

Francis, D (1995) Reflective journal: a window to preservice teachers' practical knowledge, *Teaching and Teacher Education*, **11** (3), pp 229–41

Fulwiler, T (1986) Seeing with journals, *The English Record*, **32** (3), pp 6–9

Fulwiler, T (1987) *The Journal Book*, Heinemann, Portsmouth, NH

Gatlin, L (1987) Losing control and liking it: journals in Victorian literature, in *The Journal Book*, ed T Fulwiler, Heinemann, Portsmouth, NH

Ghaye, A and Lillyman, S (1997) *Learning Journals and Critical Incidents*, Quay Books, Dinton

Gibbs, G (1988) *Learning by Doing, a guide to teaching and learning methods*, SCED, Birmingham

Griffiths, M and Tann, S (1992) Using reflective practice to link personal and public theories, *Journal of Education for Teaching*, **18** (11), pp 69–83

Grumbacher, J (1987) How writing helps physics students become better problem solvers, in *The Journal Book*, ed T Fulwiler, Heinemann, Portsmouth, NH

Grumet, M (1987) The politics of personal knowledge, *Curriculum Inquiry*, **17** (13), pp 319–35

Grumet, M (1989) Generations: reconceptualist curriculum theory and teacher education, *Journal of Teacher Education*, Jan–Feb, pp 13–17

Grumet, M (1990) Retrospective – autobiography and the analysis of educational experience, *Cambridge J Ed*, **20** (3), pp 321—5

Habermas, J (1971) *Knowledge and Human Interests*, Heinemann, London

Hadwin, A and Winne, P (1996) Study strategies have meager support. A review with recommendations for implementation, *Journal of Higher Education*, **67** (6), pp 1–17

Hahnemann, B (1986) Journal writing: a way to promoting critical thinking in nursing students, *J. Nursing Education*, **25** (5), pp 213–15

Hallberg, F (1987) Journal writing as person-making, in *The Journal Book*, ed T. Fulwiler, Heinemann, Portsmouth, NH

Handley, P (1998) Personal communication

Hartley, J (1998) *Learning and Studying*, Routledge, London

Harvey, L and Knight, P (1996) *Transforming Higher Education*, SRHE/OUP, Buckingham

Hatton, N and Smith, D (1995) Reflection in teacher education – towards definition and implementation, *Teaching and Teacher Education*, **11** (1), pp 33–49

HEA, HEBS, HPW, HPANI (1995) *Handbook on the Development of Foundation Courses in Health Promotion*, Health Promotion Wales, Cardiff

Heath, H (1998) Keeping a reflective practice diary: a practical guide, *Nurse Education Today*, **18** (18), pp 592–98

Hettich, P (1976) The journal, an autobiographical approach to learning, *Teaching of Psychology*, **3** (2), pp 60–61

Hettich, P (1980) The evaluator's journal, *CEDR Quarterly*, **13** (2), pp 19–22

Hettich, P (1988) Journal writing: an autobiographical approach to learning, *High School Psychology Teacher*, **19** (3), pp 416–17

Hettich, P (1990) Journal writing: old fare or nouvelle cuisine?, *Teaching of Psychology*, **17** (1), pp 36–39

Hickman, K (1987) There's a place for the log in the office, in *The Journal Book*, ed T Fulwiler, Heinemann, Portsmouth, NH

Holly, M (1989) Reflective writing and the spirit of inquiry, *Cambridge J of Education*, **19** (1), pp 71–80

Holly, M (1991) *Keeping a Personal-Professional Journal*, Deakin University Press, Victoria

Holly, M and McLoughlin, C (1989) *Perspectives on Teacher Professional Development*, Falmer Press, London

Hoover, L (1994) Reflective writing as a window on pre-service teachers' thought processes, *Teaching and Teacher Education*, **10**, pp 83–93

Houghton, P (1998) *Learning from Work*, Module workbook CD2006, University of Central Lancashire

Hunt, D (1987) *Beginning with Ourselves*, Brookline Books, Cambridge, MA

Jacobson, A (www) Essential learning skills across the curriculum, Oregon State Department of Education, http://snow.utoronto.ca/uploaded-files/ctr&wex.htm

Jakins, H (1970) *Fundamentals of Co-Counselling*, revised edn, Rational Island, Washington

James, C (1993) Developing reflective practice skills – the potential, Paper presented to 'The Power of the Portfolio' Conference

James, C and Denley, P (1993) Using records of experience in an undergraduate certificate in education course, *Evaluation and Research in Education 1993*, pp 23–37

Jensen, E (1979) Student journals in the social problems course: applying sociological concepts, Paper presented at the annual meeting of the Pacific Sociological Association

Jensen, V (1987) Writing in college physics, in *The Journal Book*, ed T. Fulwiler, Heinemann, Portsmouth, NH

Johns, C (1994) Nuances of reflection, *Journal of Clinical Nursing*, **3**, pp 71–75

Joyce, M (www) Double entry journals and learning logs, http://www.umcs.maine.edu/~orono/collaborative/spring/doub.html

Jung, C (1961) *Memories, Dreams and Reflections*, Random House, New York

Kaiser, R (1981) The way of the journal, *Psychology Today*, March, pp 64–76

Kelly, G (1955) *The Psychology of Personal Construct Theory*, Norton, New York

Kent, O (1987) Student journals and the goals of philosophy, in *The Journal Book*, ed T. Fulwiler, Heinemann, Portsmouth, NH

King, P and Kitchener, K (1994) *Developing Reflective Judgement*, Jossey-Bass, San Francisco

Kneale, P (1997) The rise of the 'strategic student': how can we cope?, in *Facing up to Radical Changes in Universities and Colleges*, ed M Armstrong, G Thompson and S Brown, SEDA/Kogan Page, London

Knowles, J (1993) Life history accounts as mirrors: a practical avenue for the conceptualization of reflection in teacher education, in *Conceptualizing Development in Teacher Education*, ed J Calderhead and P Gates, Falmer Press, London

Kolb, D (1984) *Experiential Learning as the Science of Learning and Development*, Prentice Hall, Englewood Cliffs, NJ

Korthagan, F (1988) The influence of learning orientation on the development of reflective teaching, in *Teachers' Professional Learning*, ed J Calderhead, Falmer Press, London

Landeen, J, Byrne, C and Brown, B (1992) 'Journal keeping as an educational strategy in learning psychiatric nursing', *Journal of Advanced Nursing*, **17**, pp 347–55

Lindberg, G (1987) The journal conference: from dialectic to dialogue, in *The Journal Book*, ed T Fulwiler, Heinemann, Portsmouth, NH

Lowenstein, S (1987) A brief history of journal keeping, in *The Journal Book*, ed T Fulwiler, Heinemann, Portsmouth, NH

Lukinsky, J (1990) Reflective withdrawal through journal writing, in *Fostering Critical Reflection in Adulthood*, ed J Mezirow, Jossey-Bass, San Francisco

Macrorie, K (1970) *Uptake*, Hayden Book Company, Rochelle Pk, NJ

Mallon, T (1984) *A Book of One's Own: People and their Diaries*, Ticknor and Fields, New York

Martin, J (1998) Personal communication

Marton, F, Hounsell, D and Entwistle, N (1997) *The Experience of Learning*, Academic Press, Edinburgh

Mayher, J, Lester, N and Pradl, M (1983) *Learning to Write, Writing to Learn*, Boynton/Cook, Upper Montclair, NJ

McCrindle, A and Christensen, C (1995) The impact of learning journals on metacognitive processes and learning performance, *Learning and Instruction*, **5** (3), pp 167–85

McManus, J (1986) Live case study, journal record in adolescent psychology, *Teaching of Psychology*, **13**, pp 70–4

Meese, G (1987) Focused leaning in chemistry research: Suzanne's journal, in *The Journal Book*, ed T Fulwiler, Heinemann, Portsmouth, NH

Miller, J (1983) A search for congruence: influence of past and present in future teachers' concepts about teaching writing, *English Education*, 15 February, pp 5–16

Miller, J (1987), Teacher's emerging texts: the empowering potential of writing in service, in *Educating Teachers*, ed J Smyth, Falmer Press, London

Miller, S (1979) Keeping a psychological journal, *The Gifted Child Quarterly*, **23**, pp 168–75

Milner, M (1957) *On Not Being Able to Paint*, Heinemann, London

Milner, M (1987) *Eternity's Sunrise: A Way of Keeping a Diary*, Virago, London

Moon, J (1996a) What can you do in a day? Advice on developing short training courses on promoting health, *Journal of the Inst. of Health Promotion*, **34** (1), pp 20–23

Moon, J (1996b) Generic level descriptors and their place in the standards debate, *In Focus*, Autumn, pp 64–69

Moon, J (1999a) *Reflection in Learning and Professional Development*, Kogan Page, London

Moon, J (1999b) Describing higher education: some conflicts and conclusions, in *Benchmarking and Threshold Standards in Higher Education*, ed H Smith, M Armstrong and S Brown, SEDA/Kogan Page, London

Moon, J and England, P (1994) The development of a highly structured workshop in health promotion, *Journal of the Institute of Health Education*, **32** (2), pp 41–44

Morgan, N and Saxon, S (1991) *Teaching Questioning and Learning*, Routledge, London

Morrison, K (1990) *Learning Logs*, Department of Education, University of Durham, Durham

Morrison, K (1996) Developing reflective practice in higher degree students through a learning journal, *Studies in HE*, **21** (3), pp 317–32

Mortimer, J (1998) Motivating student learning through facilitating independence: self and peer assessment of reflective practice – an action research project, in *Motivating Students*, ed S Brown, S Armstrong and G Thompson, SEDA/Kogan Page, London

Mülhaus, S and Löschmann, M (1997) Improving independent learning with aural German programmes, in *Flexible Learning in Action*, ed R Hudson, S Maslin-Prothero and L Oates, SEDA/Kogan Page, London

Neary, M (1998) Personal communication

Newman, D (www) Project learning journals, http://143.117.143.9/mgt/itsoc/proj/learjour.html

NICEC (1998) Developing career management skills in higher education, Briefing, Nat. Inst. For Careers Education and Counselling, Sheraton House, Castle Pk, Cambridge

NCIHE (1997) *Report of National Inquiry into Higher Education (The Dearing Report)*, NCIHE

November, P (1993) Journals for the journey into deep learning, *Research and Development in HE*, **16**, pp 299–303

Oberg, A and Underwood, S (1992) Facilitative self development – reflections on experience,' in *Understanding Teacher Development*, ed A Hargreaves and M Fulton, Teacher's College Press, New York

Oliver, R (1998) Personal communication

Paris, S and Winograd, P (1990) How metacognition can promote academic learning and instruction, in *Dimensions of Thinking and Cognitive Instruction*, ed B Jones and L Idol, Lawrence Erlbaum, Hillsdale, NJ

Parker, R and Goodkin, V (1987) *The Consequences of Writing: enhancing learning in the disciplines*, Boynton/Cook, NJ

Parnell, J (1998) Personal communication

Paul, R (1990) Critical and reflective thinking. A philosophical perspective, in *Dimensions of Thinking and Cognitive Instruction*, ed B Jones and L Idol, Lawrence Erlbaum Associates, Hillsdale, NJ

Paulson, T, Paulson, P and Meyer, C (1991) What makes a portfolio a portfolio?, *Educational Leadership,* February, pp 60–65

Perry, W (1970) *Forms of Intellectual and Academic Developments in College Years*, Holt, Rhinehart and Winston, New York

Piaget, J (1971) *Biology and Knowledge*, Edinburgh University Press, Edinburgh

Pinar, W (1975) Currere: towards reconceptualization, in *Curriculum Theorizing*, ed W Pinar, McCutcham Publishing Corp., Berkeley, CA

Prawat, R (1989) Promoting access to knowledge, strategy and disposition in students: a research synthesis', *Review of Educational Research*, **50** (1), pp 1–41

Prawat, R (1991) Conversations with self and settings, *American Educational Research Journal*, **28** (4), pp 737–57

Progoff, I (1975) *At a Journal Workshop*, Dialogue House Library, New York

Progoff, I (1980) *The Practice of Process Meditation*, Dialogue House Library, New York

Rainer, T (1978) *The New Diary. How to use a journal for self guidance and extended creativity*, J P Tarcher Inc, Los Angeles

Redwine, M (1989) The autobiography as a motivating factor for students, in *Making Sense of Experiential Learning*, ed S Warner Weil and I McGill, SRHE/OUP, Buckingham

Reid, A and Leigh, E (1998) Three dimensional images in self assessment of learning, Paper presented at Improving Student Learning Conference, Brighton University, September

Richardson, L (1994) Writing. A method of inquiry, in *Handbook of Qualitative Research*, ed N Denzil and Y Lincoln, Sage, London

Richardson, V (1997) Constructiveness teaching and teacher education: theory and practice, in *Constructivist Teacher Education*, ed V Richardson, Falmer Press, London

Roderick, J (1986) Dialogue journal writing: context for reflecting on self as teacher and researcher, *J Curr and Supervision*, **1** (4), pp 305–15

Roderick, J and Berman, L (1984) Dialoguing and dialogue journals, *Language Arts*, **61** (7), pp 686–92

Rogers, C (1969) *Freedom to Learn*, Charles E. Merrill, Columbus, OH

Ross, D (1989) First steps in developing a reflective approach, *Journal of Teacher Education*, **40** (2), pp 22–30

Rovegno, I (1992) Learning to reflect on teaching; a case study of one preservice physical education teacher, *The Elementary School Journal*, **92** (4), pp 491–510

Sagor, R (1991) What project LEARN reveals about corroborative action research, *Educational Leadership*, March, pp 6–9

Salisbury, J (1994) *Becoming Qualified – an ethnography of a post-experience teacher-training course*, PhD thesis, University College of Wales, Cardiff

Sanford, B (1988) Writing reflectively, *Language Arts*, **65** (7), pp 652–57

Schneider, M and Killick, J (1998) *Writing for Self Discovery*, Element Books, Shaftsbury, Dorset

Schön, D (1983) *The Reflective Practitioner*, Jossey-Bass, San Francisco

Schön, D (1987) *Educating the Reflective Practitioner*, Jossey-Bass, San Francisco

Selfe, C and Arbabi, F (1986) Writing to learn – Engineering students journals, in *Writing Across the Disciplines*, ed A Young and T Fulwiler, Boynton/Cook, Upper Montclair, NJ

Selfe, C, Petersen, B and Nahrgang, C (1986) Journal writing in mathematics, in *Writing Across the Disciplines*, ed A Young and T Fulwiler, Boynton/Cook, Upper Montclair, NJ

Smyth, J (1987) *Changing the Nature of Pedagogical Knowledge*, Falmer Press, Lewes

Smyth, J (1989) Developing and sustaining critical reflection in teacher education, *J Teacher Education*, **40** (2), pp 2–9

Shohet, R (1985) *Dream Sharing*, Turnstone Press, Wellingborough, Northants

Sparkes-Langer, G and Colton, A (1991) Synthesis of research on teachers' reflective thinking, *Educational Leadership*, March, pp 37–44

Sparkes-Langer, G, Simmons, J, Pasch, M, Colton, A and Starko, A (1990) Reflective pedagogical thinking: how can we promote and measure it?, *Journal of Teacher Education*, **41**, pp 23–32

Staton J (1998) Contributions of the dialogue journal research to communicating, thinking and learning in J Staton, S Peyton and J Reed (eds) (1998) *Dialogue Journal Communication*, Ablex, Norwood, NJ

Staton, J, Shuy, R, Peyton, S and Reed, L (eds) (1988) *Dialogue Journal Communication*, Ablex, Norwood, NJ

Steffens, H (1987) Journals in the teaching of history, in *The Journal Book*, ed T. Fulwiler, Heinemann, Portsmouth, NH

Stephani, L (1997) Reflective teaching in higher education, *UCOSDA Briefing Paper* 42, UCoSDA, Sheffield

Stephani, L (*THES*, April 16th 1999) Reflections on Self Control

Storr, A (1988) *Solitude*, Flamingo Press, London

Sumsion, J and Fleet, A (1996) Reflection: can we assess it? Should we assess it?, *Assessment and Evaluation in HE*, **21** (2), pp 121–30

Surbeck, E, Han, E and Moyer, J (1991) Assessing reflective responses in journals, *Educational Leadership*, March, pp 25–27

Tama, C and Peterson, K (1991) Achieving reflectivity through literature, *Educational Leadership*, March, pp 22–4

Terry, W (1984) A 'forgetting' journal' for memory courses, *Teaching of Psychology*, **11**, pp 111–12

Tripp, D (1987) Teacher's journals and collaborative research, in *Changing the Nature of Pedagogical Knowledge*, ed J Smyth, Falmer Press, Lewes

Van Manen, M (1977) Linking ways of knowing and ways of being, *Curriculum Inquiry*, **6**, pp 205–08

Van Rossum, E and Schenk, S (1984) The relationship between learning conception, study strategy and learning outcome, *British Journal of Educational Psychology*, **54**, pp 73–83

Voss, M, (1988) The light at the end of the journal: a teacher learns about learning, *Language Arts*, **65** (7), pp 669–74

Vygotsky, L (1978) *Mind in Society: the Development of Higher Psychological Processes*, Harvard University Press, Cambridge, MA

Wagenaar, T (1984) Using student journals in sociology courses, *Teaching Sociology*, **11**, pp 419–37

Walker, D (1985) Writing and reflection, in *Reflection: Turning Experience into Learning*, ed D Boud, R Keogh and D Walker, Kogan Page, London

Wedman, J and Martin, M (1986) Exploring the development of reflective thinking through journal writing, *Reading Improvement*, **23** (1), pp 68–71

Weil, S (1996) From the other side of science: new possibilities for dialogue in academic writing, *Changes*, **3**, pp 223–31

Weinstein, C (1987) Fostering learning autonomy through the use of learning strategies, *J Reading*, **7**, pp 590–95

Wellington, B (1991) The promise of reflective practice, *Educational Leadership*, March, pp 4–5

Wetherell, J, and Mullins, G (1996) The use of student journals in problem-based learning, *Medical Education*, 30, pp 105–11

Wetherell, J and Mullins, G (www) Drilling for gold, http://web.acue.adelaide.edu.au/leap/focus/pbl/wetherell.html

Wildman, T and Niles, J (1987) Reflective teachers, tensions between abstractions and realities, *Journal of Teacher Education*, **3**, pp 25–31

Winitzky, N and Kauchak, D (1997) Constructivism in teacher education: applying cognitive theory to teacher learning, in *Constructivist Teacher Education*, ed V Richardson, Falmer Press, London

Wolf, J (1980) Experiential learning in professional education: concepts and tools, *New Directions for Experiential Learning*, **8**, pp 1–26

Wolf, M (1989) Journal writing: a means to an end in educating students to work with older adults, *Gerontology and Geriatrics Education*, **10**, pp 53–62

Wolf Moondance (1994) *Rainbow Medicine*, Sterling Publishing Co, New York

Wolf, V (1978) *A Writer's Diary*, Triad, Granada, London

Woods, P (1987) Life histories and teacher knowledge, in *Educating Teachers – Changing the Nature of Pedagogical Knowledge*, ed J Smyth, Falmer Press, Lewes

Yinger, R (1985) Journal writing as a learning tool, *The Volta Review*, **87** (5), pp 21–33

Yinger, R and Clark, M (1981) Reflective journal writing: theory and practice, *Occasional Paper* No 50, East Lansing, Michigan State University Inst. for Research on Teaching

Young, A and Fulwiler, T (1986) *Writing across the Disciplines*, Boynton/Cook, Upper Montclair, NJ

Index